Aging Beyond Belief

Don Ardell

69 tips
for REAL wellness

Reason
Exuberance
And
Liberty

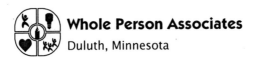

Whole Person Associates
Duluth, Minnesota

Whole Person Associates
210 West Michigan Street
Duluth, MN 55802-1908

800-247-6789

books@wholeperson.com
www.wholeperson.com

Aging Beyond Belief
69 Tips for REAL Wellness: Reason, Exuberance, And Liberty

Printed in the United States of America

10 9 8 7 6 5 4 3 2 1

Editorial Director: Carlene Sippola
Art Director: Joy Morgan Dey

Library of Congress Control Number: 2007929032
ISBN: 978-1-57025-220-4

Dedication

To my grandchildren Madison (4), Cadence (2),
Charlie (2) and Buddy Miles (1). It's never too late, or too
soon, to start aging under the influence—of a **REAL** wellness
lifestyle. Of course, by the time they can read this book, such
patterns will be well established, thanks to their parents
Sara and Josh, Jeanne and Steve, and Jon and Staci.

To my darling wife Carol, who reads and improves
all my stuff. I am fortunate to be aging under the influence
of a beautiful and athletic companion whose wellness lifestyle
influences my own every day.

To Bob Ludlow, a former cycling buddy
and lifelong friend who serves as an unofficial editor-in-chief
and part-time director of my continuing education.
He provides near-daily streams of articles, political
cartoons, book recommendations and, best of all, personal
commentaries on current events.

To Judd Allen, Rick Clark, Grant Donovan, Bill Hettler,
Lenore Howe, Steve Jonas, Sandy Scott and Wendy Shore,
all of whom made invaluable contributions to these tips
and to the essays that appear daily at SeekWellness.com and
in the weekly ARDELL WELLNESS REPORTS.

Finally, kudos to Carlene, Peg and Joy at Whole Person for
skillful editing, patience, tolerance and skillful design.

Preface

REAL is used in this book as an acronym for three amazing lifestyle qualities. These qualities are key, in my view, to a life that is healthier, more enjoyable and ever so much more satisfying than what passes for "normal," which is not very healthy,enjoyable or satisfying. The REAL qualities I offer are Reason, Exuberance And Liberty. These qualities are foundation elements in 69 tips for genuine, authentic and yes, REAL wellness!

The wellness concept is a powerful idea. It's a term that has been widely used, but the best parts of the original wellness mindset or philosophy have been neglected. These elements include personal responsibility, critical thinking, the quest for added meaning and purpose, humor, play, happiness and emotional intelligence. Make no mistake—there is a lot more to REAL wellness than exercise and nutrition. All parts or skill areas of REAL wellness are addressed in the 69 tips. These tips will demonstrate that REAL wellness is not a product, a healing remedy, a medical service or anything else outside of oneself, but a way of life that you manage and direct. You can't buy pills or treatments for REAL wellness—it's a mindset and lifestyle you control. Therefore, let Reason, Exuberance And Liberty—REAL wellness, be your guide!

In these tips, you will find a lot of advice for aging well. The tips are based upon your willingness and ability to employ reason (evidence-based decision-making) in order to experience exuberance in daily life that in turn will enrich your enjoyment of maximum liberty (freedom and choice). That kind of wellness, gentle reader, is the genuine number, the real McCoy—it's nothing less than REAL wellness. That's the idea of this book. I'm confident you'll find it so.

In short, this book applies the term wellness to personal responsibility, exercise and fitness, nutrition, stress management and meaning and purpose. It celebrates reason as critical thinking and exuberant aliveness, joy and pleasure in a context of maximum liberty, choice and freedom. And all this is just for starters. I don't want to limit the use of the term! REAL wellness invites attention as well to sound relationships, resilience and much else that we associate with a high quality of life, not just related to aging—but in all stages of life.

Thirty years after the publication of my first book *High Level Wellness: An Alternative To Doctors, Drugs and Disease* (Rodale, 1977; Bantam, 1979; Ten Speed Press, 1987), this book about aging well represents a celebration of the wellness concept, at its best. REAL wellness represents the way I celebrate and communicate the concept. That is what I have intended with the 69 tips for aging under the influence of a healthy and satisfying lifestyle. I hope you enjoy and find these tips helpful in shaping your own aging process. After all, if you're going to age anyway, why not do so along wellness lines? REAL wellness lines.

Introduction

Aging. Getting older, slowing down, the autumn years. Not something any of us would choose for the discounts, if we could stay 39 for another year or, better yet, half a dozen more decades. But, aging happens. We all do it, until the final curtain call. Signs and symptoms of aging creep into our awareness sometime around age 40. I myself am rumored to be approaching senior-hood. Just the other day, I thought I saw a sign of aging in my barely noticeable receding hairline. However, considering I'm only 69, I doubt anyone else noticed, yet. But I'm aware of it—and that's what matters.

The question is—what of it? Should you struggle, resist, deny, and invest in repairs and restorations? Or, is it better to just give up and resign yourself to a gradual fade—into oblivion or Valhalla? Neither—this is a false dichotomy, a too-narrow choice. You can do something else. You can age under the influence—of a wellness lifestyle. Welcome to this, a guided tour of tips for aging healthfully and well with maximum life enjoyment along the way.

I've been pondering, experimenting and writing tips for "aging under the influence" (AUI) of a wellness lifestyle for many years. For this book, I condensed decades of wellness advice-giving into 69 distinct tidbits of guidance for intelligently designing your own evolution. Yes, you can organize your thinking and behavior to evolve into the all-around fittest you possible.

I selected 69 suggestions for AUI based upon the idea that I ought to have one tip for each year of my existence. I hope you find many of these tips highly useful, as well as interesting and provocative.

Feel free to write me with additional tips, if you think of any. They could be helpful if I get much older.

Objectives

If you plan to age, you will enjoy the later years more if you AUI of a wellness lifestyle. Doing so will enable the best possible health, the highest available energy levels, the greatest obtainable degree of physical mobility and the fullest mental capacities. Furthermore, from the perspective of non-positive but still important payoffs, AUI should prove highly beneficial because you will minimize the downside risks or disabilities of aging. AUI of a wellness lifestyle will save money (e.g., you won't need as many medications and medical interventions as your peers), minimize pain (fewer illnesses and failed parts) and maybe you will last longer—no guarantees, as random chance plays a big role in longevity. However, you will at least boost your odds of a longer life. But the best reason is pure pleasure—you will enjoy yourself more the remaining days of your life. These should be viewed as the true wonder years, the best of all your times.

Thus there are both attractive objectives of a positive (enjoyable) and negative (avoidance) nature that favor devoting serious attention to these 69 tips for AUI. Make a conscious choice to do so—and thereby make the latter decades as fulfilling and delightful as possible.

Caveats

The tips are designed to stimulate your creative adaptations, not as blueprints. That should be obvious but you never know—some folks take everything way too seriously. Not all tips will work for everyone—that's why there are so many! If just one tips changes your life in a significant way, this book will be great value. Some tips may seem like terrible ideas to some readers (e.g., see tip # 11—definitely not for everybody). Of course, all the tips make sense to me. You may find some of them a little "out there" or maybe too timid—tastes are widely different. In any event, the tips are consistent with my experiences. Each one seems just the thing for AUI, but it's best that you interpret all of them to suit your style, tastes and peculiar inclinations.

And one more thing—don't worry; there are no tips that I myself do not follow. These are tested by my experience as a wellness enthusiast nearly all of my adult years. They are also based, to the extent possible, on science and reason! I have not "channeled" these tips from any 16th century mystics (e.g., Nostradamus), nor have any been delivered on a space ship—just for me. Nor are other amazing revelations at play here. The focus on science and reason is vital in health-related works and everything else, in my opinion. Therefore, I made every effort to ensure that the tips are consistent with studies—and referenced the studies and other sources for your perusal. It's true—I made up the tips themselves, but I had a lot of help from many bright people who know how aging works from studying the phenomenon over many years in controlled ways.

I have not included any aging tips I find personally unattractive, even if some experts think they could add a few years to your life. An example is calorie restriction. There is no tip in this book to the effect that you should starve yourself in order to live longer. If doing so were a sure thing for added years (highly unlikely), I still would not recommend it. Don't look for any really bizarre life extension notions in these tips, such as inhaling virgins' breath, eating gold or implanting monkey glands. I'm guessing you are quite relieved to know that.

On that parting introductory note, here are my 69 tips. Let's get started. Enjoy.

The Tips

Much has been written about the nature, principles and applications of a term made popular in just the past couple decades called "wellness." Nobody is authorized to make the rules of what it is and what it isn't, but that is not to say someone ought not to step forward to give it a try. I volunteer.

I began writing about wellness in the 1970s. I was the director of a health planning agency in the San Francisco Bay Area at the time I started learning about a wide range of ideas and principles that would shape what became a modest movement within and then well beyond the medical system. Our planning organization and others like it in metropolitan areas around the country was designed by committees of politicians and health experts over several years to improve health status and to bring order to the health care system.

Alas, two prominent factors kept such agencies from being effective: 1) We had almost no authority, so medical leaders and others who were supposed to be guided by our work paid little attention to the plans we devised for coordinated health care facilities and services; and 2) We were going about it the wrong way. We were trying to change the way the medical system worked. Even if we had succeeded we would not have succeeded! We did not recognize at the time that the way to promote health and save costs was to inform, motivate, convince, inspire, guide and otherwise support people to take better care of themselves and rely less on the medical system.

From this realization came a period of reflection on my part that prompted a career change—from health planner administrator to doctoral candidate and, a few years later, to a life as a writer, lecturer and consultant promoting wellness. To this day, 30 years after publication of my book *High Level Wellness: An Alternative to Doctors,*

Drugs and Disease (Rodale Press), I believe the wellness concept, if it is the REAL wellness concept, is the most promising approach available to society and to you to boost health status AND save medical costs.

During the formative years of wellness in the 70s and 80s, there were a good number of conferences and seminars, policy papers, scholarly articles, books and so on devoted to the concept that eventually morphed into a wellness movement. Not surprisingly, the wellness concept was given a slightly different spin by nearly everyone who came into contact with it. To this day, variations abound.

What follows is my idea of a wellness mindset, translated into terms suited to everyone who wants to age well. In my view, wellness should be an evidence based mindset geared to high levels of well-being and life satisfaction. I believe such a lifestyle is associated with countless benefits, if given half a chance. My advice—learn about what wellness can be for you, at it's best, and don't even think about aging without it.

Let me mention a few key ideas about wellness and a number of wonderful benefits to get things started.

Wellness is positive. The focus is not on hazards and risks, but rather on satisfactions and pleasures. It is comprehensive, not about just fitness, nutrition and managing stress but also entails critical thinking, humor and play, emotional intelligence and the quest for added meaning and purpose in life—and much more, which I'll highlight in these tips. It is based on science and reason, not New Age wishful thinking or reliance or even inclusion of "alternative" or other therapies, modalities or healing systems. It is also a mindset or philosophy founded on personal responsibility and accountability. There is more, as you will learn in the coming 68 tips.

Six benefits that I find especially appealing about real wellness are:

1. Better health.
A wellness lifestyle boosts energy while lowering risks of illness.

2. Better appearance.
You'll look thinner and fitter, even more interesting, if you follow such a lifestyle.

3. Better sex.
Unclogged arteries facilitate blood flow to all body parts.

4. Better decisions.
You develop a greater desire for reason and science, sound evidence and other critical thinking skills associated with genuine maturity.

5. Better role model.
In non-verbal ways (e.g., style/appearance and value commitments) you convey a superior message to your impressionable relatives and others.

6. Better perspectives.
Some things are important and deserve a lot of energy, but most are not a big deal. Finding satisfying, energizing meaning and purpose in life, for example—now that's important. Dealing with little vexations, silly people, worries about things you can't change—not so important.

Naturally, it is better to be young than old, other things being the same, which they never are, just as it's better to be rich than poor, fit than fat and alive than dead. But, so what? As noted in the chorus of John Prine's immortal Dear Abby, "You have no complaint—You are what your are and you ain't what you ain't." Not so grammatical, but so very true.

Aging is not always pleasant but, like gravity and evolution, it's more than a theory. It's part of life, at least for everyone fortunate enough to attain such status.

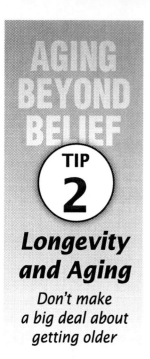

AGING BEYOND BELIEF

TIP 2

Longevity and Aging

Don't make a big deal about getting older

*E*verybody does it, it can't be avoided and there is no cure. Each day is an opportunity to enjoy being younger than you ever will be again, so think and act as vigorously and with as much exuberance as you can muster. Billions are spent annually to slow or, more often, disguise the inevitable markers of aging. Such a waste. All this is futile. As Ecclesiastes would say, "a vanity of vanities, an incomparable excess." I personally have a soft spot for excess, but not to the point of being incomparably self-delusional about my vanities.

"Want in on a little health secret? Move to Canada. An impressive array of data shows that Canadians live longer, healthier lives than we do. What's more, they pay roughly half as much per capita Americans ($2,163 versus $4,887 in 2001) for the privilege." (*Los Angeles Times*, February 23, 2004).

Did you know there's a mathematical formula that predicts maximal age? There is—and the formula is the basis for the agreed-upon maximum human age being set at 120. (This means I could be writing a second edition to this book in the year 2058.) The formula for maximal age is six times the number of years from birth to biological maturity. Humans take about 20 years to reach maturity, so multiply that by six and there it is—a 120-year limit. (The oldest well-documented age ever was 122.)

Remember, many factors affect longevity, particularly lifestyle choices (e.g., exercise, diet), personality, social life and genetics. Approximately "one-third of aging is heritable, the rest is acquired—that means you are responsible for your own old age." (Tara Parker-Pope, "What Science Tells Us About Growing Older—And Staying Healthy," *Wall Street Journal*, June 20, 2005; Page R1.)

Longevity in this country is nothing to cheer about. When compared with other Western nations, the U.S. is doing worse now than 50 years ago! We are currently losing ground, not making longevity advances, relative to other countries. This might surprise you. Yes, we live longer but our relative position is poorer compared with comparable societies than it was when Eisenhower was president. This despite our having the costliest medical care system on earth!

A World Health Organization study released last year put Canadian life expectancy at birth at 79.8 years, Japan's at 81.9 and America's at 77.3!

In 1900, the lifespan in America was 47.3. I shudder to think of all my friends who would be dead now if that figure had not improved over the course of the past century. With no advances, there would be few to no competitors in my 65-69 age group in road races, duathlons and triathlons. A similar 30-year gain in life expectancy into the future would render the average lifespan in the year 2112 a robust 107.3 years.

How might that come about? Perhaps from a wide range of social changes over time, like more nutritious foods and challenging but fun phys ed in schools, campaigns for safer sex and more effective ways to end insane behaviors, like smoking. (It will help also if humanity refrains from setting off any thermonuclear devices.)

Imagine the excitement of watching men and women in their 120s crossing finish lines at road races and multi-sport competitions, to the cheers of the multitudes, with "Rocky" music blaring from loudspeakers. It would be inspirational.

However, it's also implausible. Wellness is good, wellness is great but I still don't believe that there will be dramatic advances in phys ed in schools, better diets or other social changes. I hope I'm mistaken about this. If there were such changes and many others consistent with the spread of wellness mindsets like some positive contagion, even that might not produce really dramatic increase in lifespan, though quality boosts would be remarkable. If there are any significant increases in lifespan, the more likely impetus will be improved scientific understanding and attendant manipulation of biological aging processes. But, I'm not wildly optimistic about this scenario, either.

Nor does the U.S. Social Security Administration project dramatic gains for the next century similar to that realized over the last one. Their projections foresee life spans into the mid-80s, which is still pretty impressive. Unless, as some fear, the obesity epidemic gets worse.

In any event, getting older is not such a big deal if you stay younger than nearly everyone else your age! The remaining tips will offer plenty of ideas for doing just that.

*P*ace yourself in learning about wellness. Create a more supportive network to live this way. Create a wellness support network, over time. Don't rush it. Pace yourself. Consider attending a workshop in your area, or a seminar or lecture dealing with aspects of better living that you find appealing. Check out the program first, since the word "wellness" is often misapplied. Sometimes, it's used as a marketing gimmick with little understanding of the unique qualities of the concept. You would not want to inadvertently attend a program billed as a wellness event, only to be pitched to invest in a multi-level sales organization for vitamin-fortified seaweed, or something equally bizarre having no remote connection with a wellness lifestyle.

A Discovery Process

Pace yourself in learning about wellness

Here's a specific suggestion: Check out the National Wellness Conference. It is a festival by and for wellness seekers and promoters held annually in Stevens Point, Wisconsin. It's not entirely focused on aging, but everything about the wellness concept can be readily applied to AUI. I'm quite an enthusiast of the event myself—I have been attending the weeklong gatherings for over 25 years. Check out the NWI website at www.nationalwellness.org. You could also call (800) 243-8694 or send an E-mail. One way or another, ask to be placed on the mailing list for the free annual program sent worldwide in the spring.

An important part of creating a supportive culture is understanding your current support system. Take a close, conscious look at the norms, customs and rituals that shaped and guided your formative years. Think about how pervasive yet subtle these norms and customs and traditions were and how, little by little and bit-by-bit, you digested it all during the early years. Identify those traditions that today, after a lifetime, are more like obstacles than cherished values, and set yourself free from anything now seen as nonsense, dogma, clichés and platitudes. These are enemies of your capacity for reason leading to excellence. These are obstacles to more supportive networks that will make your best possible life much more attainable.

Do you know what "central processing unit" (CPU) I'm talking about? I mean the one in your head containing 100 billion neurons, the one able to make about 1,000 trillion interconnections or so, according to R. Grant Steen in *The Evolving Brain* (Prometheus Books, Amherst, NY, 2007). Your brain, neurophysiologist Steen suggests, is "arguably the most complex object in the universe." The more you learn about consciousness and unconsciousness, learning, memory, the role of genes, motivation, aggression and even your brain's evolution, the more you will look after it. That is, give it new data, use it wisely and take good care of the rest of the organism to which it is attached.

Understanding the Aging Brain

Learn as much as you can about your own CPU

All this attention to the brain takes on added significance as the years accrue on the old CPU. The CPUs in computers can be replaced, but the one in your skull has to be upgraded, regularly if not automatically. There's work involved, which is often the case when worthwhile returns are at issue. It's just one more "cross to bear" (I prefer "responsibility to assume") associated with "senior-hood." While it tempting to conclude that there is not much (good) to be said for getting older, consider this before getting discouraged:

- We're wiser than we were as youths.

- We have more money.

- We're not as obsessed with sex. (This is a rumor.)

- We have time-tested ideas about the great existential questions. (They are most likely peculiar, twisted and irrational like mine, but if they help you make sense of things and live a good life, who cares?)

- We feel better about ourselves.

- We don't have to support our children.

Besides, what's there not to like about getting older given the fact that it's not optional for anyone partial to breathing?

Of course, not all the assertions I listed apply in every case; in some codgers, none applies. I believe it was H. L. Mencken who said, "The older I grow the more I distrust the familiar doctrine that age brings wisdom."

New evidence has come to light suggesting that Mencken SHOULD have placed more trust in that familiar doctrine. It might, happily enough, be mostly true.

The latest research suggests that, with regard to older brains, like mine, there's good news and bad news. The bad is not even that bad. Sure, old brains process information more slowly and less nimbly, so decisions (e.g., whether to drive left or right, stop or pull over) take longer. This is a bit of a problem when, for instance, a fast-moving Hummer is being managed by an old brain. But, the good news more than makes up for the pokey decision-making, provided you get where you're going in one piece without leaving a trail of carnage behind you. It's true that old brains are not as good at "multitasking" as they once were.

But, here's the good news, according to Marilyn Albert of Johns Hopkins School of Medicine, where brain studies on aging have been getting a lot of attention. (See "Old Brains Don't Work That Badly After All, Especially Trained Ones," *The Wall Street Journal*, March 3, 2006; Page B1.) "Neurons don't abandon ship." Our brains retain the ingredients needed, IF we continue to use them and keep the rest of the body in tune. This brings to mind another old adage, "You can live to be a hundred if you give up all things that make you want to live to be a hundred." This adage is wrong, according to the new findings. You, particularly your brain functions, will live longer if you DON'T give up the things that make you want to live to be a hundred.

Want to have a "fit brain" with high-end neural circuitry when you're old? Exercise—both your body AND your mind, daily—and don't slack off in the later years.

Here is a summary of some of the latest findings:

- Even 70-year-olds produce new neurons as well as keeping the old ones needed for memory (hippocampus region) and planning and judgment (frontal cortex).

- While a rose is a rose is a rose, neurons are different in different older folks. A geezer who does not employ his/her brain with multiple new experiences, who does not stay physically fit, socially engaged and active in complex environments will NOT have the neuron health of a wellness enthusiast who meets all these standards.

- The epicenter of the brain for purposes of studying neural well-being is the prefrontal cortex region. If your neurons here are "firing on all cylinders," so to speak, you will be able to pay attention to important stuff and ignore the rest.

- One study found that old brains could be trained to act like young ones by mental exercises that require the use of both hemispheres of the brain. (Results were described in the February 2006 journal *Neurobiology of Aging*.) This demonstrated that the brains of older adults could stay "relatively flexible, able to alter brain circuits in response to training."

As Hans Selye once advised, there's nothing wrong with retirement as long as it does not interfere with your work. By "work," Selye meant keeping up the social and intellectual demands, avoiding routine and staying engaged in daily affairs.

I like all these requirements. I'll end this now in order to go off looking for some daily affairs. There you have it—one more reason to live a wellness lifestyle with panache and verve.

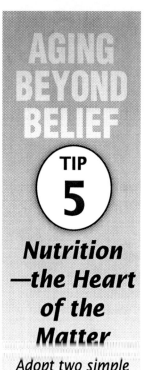

AGING BEYOND BELIEF

TIP 5

Nutrition —the Heart of the Matter

Adopt two simple nutritional goals and work to realize both

*T*his tip is supported by research done at the Agriculture and Health and Human Services Departments. The two nutritional goals are: 1) Eat fruits and vegetables on at least three separate occasions spaced throughout the day; and 2) Consume at least two cups of fruit and three cups of vegetables daily.

Another study published in the journal *Neurology* (10/24/2006), based on a six-year research project involving 4000 seniors, hinted strongly that it's never too late to gain a mental edge in this fashion. Two daily servings of vegetables—that's all it takes. What a deal.

Veggies are much cheaper than drugs and doctor visits. Besides, nobody ever got smarter medicating or seeing doctors. The seniors study just mentioned, done at the Rush Center for Healthy Aging in Chicago, suggests the two-serving daily fix slows cognitive mental declines by as much as 40 percent. This is judged the equivalent of a five-year age discount! There are not many ways to drop five years of aging effects—don't pass up such a deal!

Vegetables, particularly those in the leafy green category, provide such brain benefits because of their antioxidant compounds, such as vitamin E, flavonoids and carotenoids. What's more, the absorption of these compounds is enhanced if they are prepared using olive or vegetable oils, or other poly or mono-unsaturated fats.

Such high consumption levels will ensure that you get loads of phytonutrients—great as antioxidants that inhibit free radical cell damages and helpful, as well, in weight control. At present, 90 percent of the US population does not realize this intake standard. This partially accounts for the fact that two-thirds of Americans are overweight and 90 million suffer from chronic diseases. Naturally, our individual needs vary, depending on our exercise levels, age and sex. To personalize this tip in accord with your situation, go to www.mypyramid.gov. (For details about top-rated fruits and veggies, see "More Reasons to Eat Your Veggies," *Wall Street Journal*, 7/25/06, D1 and D3).

This tip is offered despite the general rule that you should be suspicious of claims for one specific food or another. This tip is not for a single food, but two classes of food. Still, it is useful to note that it is wise to reserve judgments. Always allow time for your critical thinking talents to come into play. Let's say someone insists that his product will increase your energy, shrink your derriere and/or grow hair on your head. What to do? My advice—be respectful and kind but don't agree or buy anything. Be skeptical. Assuming you were even mildly interested, ask for evidence. Insist that it be from a disinterested third party—and take your time before deciding.

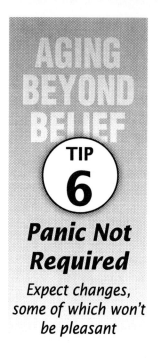

TIP

6

Panic Not Required

Expect changes, some of which won't be pleasant

*A*t first, naturally enough, many changes will look and feel like crises. This is natural, since they ARE crises (e.g., receding hairlines, wrinkles and fewer offers of leading roles in major motion pictures). Disappointment, upset and worry can't he helped—it's quite unavoidable. But, resolve not to dwell forevermore on such things. You are still younger than you are ever going to be again—make the most of it. After a short period adjusting to changes, start plotting rejuvenation, not just a recovery to a boring survival level. Think about actual advances you might attempt that will leave you better off than you were before change intervened and unsettled things.

Prepare for change by building up your level of resilience. Cultivating this quality will protect your vitality, induce added serenity and pave the way for continued passion, adaptability and optimism.

You will build and strengthen your resilience by doing positive things, like reading this book about AUI of a wellness lifestyle. There are many other ways. A few additional steps for creating increased resilience for better adaptation to change might include:

* Nurturing your network of connections with others—thus avoiding isolation.

* Helping others.

* Protecting your routines. Change, as Alvin Toffler emphasized in his 1971 megabit "Future Shock," can be tempered by safeguarding the familiar. Don't change things you don't have to while adapting to crises.

* Setting goals and picking up the pace toward accomplishing them. Fashion modest goals, at least initially, goals that are

easy to realize. Building confidence is more important for resilience than reaching the goal, at least for a while.

* Keeping the big picture in mind. Relative to all kinds of good things going your way, a crisis does not loom as large if kept in perspective.

See change for what it really is—a part of life, as inexorable as day and night, taxes and politicians who don't live up to your hopes.

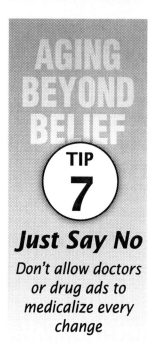

TIP

7

Just Say No

*Don't allow doctors
or drug ads to
medicalize every
change*

*T*here are limits to modern medicine, however wondrous in some ways. Not all ills need pills or treatments. Due to immense pressure from all kinds of powerful interests, particularly the drug industry and elderly lobbies, Congress has lavished $600 billion worth of prescription drug benefits for seniors via the Medicare program. While many seniors benefit from some drugs, vast numbers of the elderly are seriously overmedicated. Medical students have told me one of the first things taught in medical school is that whenever a senior presents with signs of confusion, the first thing to rule out is medications. Polypharmacy was seen a serious problem in the 1980s. Now it's much worse.

I'd like to see Congress institute a few Medicare reforms before taxpayers go broke. We have to figure out ways to promote healthier, fitter seniors so future recipients won't have to rely on Medicare benefits as so many seniors do today. I wish at least half, if not all, new Medicare funds were earmarked for promoting an AUI wellness mindset among seniors. With greater levels of personal responsibility for their own well-being, older Americans would do more to become less dependent on drugs for everyday life management.

Since older citizens have vastly more chronic conditions, they have come to rely on a cocktail of medications. These range from over-the-counter remedies, to prescription drugs to herbal supplements—not to mention a grab bag of alternative fixes wholly without any evidence base of effectiveness.

Did you know that the number of medication alerts for potential drug problems increased from 3.4 million in 1999 to 7.9 million last year? The fact that one in six seniors had at least five different doctors and filled prescriptions at five different pharmacies compromises the safety of the products. Some patients take as many as a dozen different medications, almost always without doctor's review or awareness.

The head of the California Pharmacists Association acknowledged that overmedication is a serious national problem. A story (*Idaho Press Tribune*, July 16, 2003) noted that "seniors may get one prescription from an internist and another from a rheumatologist and get each filled at the closest pharmacy, ending up with an expensive and unnecessary rainbow of little bottles on their kitchen shelf."

I think you would be better off if Congress supported wellness education for Medicare recipients and other Americans. Better to pay for elder memberships in health clubs than more medications, save for the basics that should be tightly supervised and dispensed when no other strategies will relieve pain or improve conditions. If you have any political influence, please exert it to encourage a better fix for seniors than we currently get from shortsighted political leaders.

Excessive diagnoses, brought about in part by breakthrough testing technologies (e.g., CT scans, ultrasounds, MRI and PET scans) and changed rules (e.g., lower thresholds for diabetes, hypertension, osteoporosis and obesity) have led to a situation where half the population have diseases! As noted by physician author H. Gilbert Welch, "the larger threat posed by American medicine is … an epidemic of diagnoses … But the real problem with the epidemic of diagnoses is that it leads to an epidemic of treatments." ("Too Many Diagnoses Make Us Ill," *St. Petersburg Times*, January 7, 2007, p.1)

A lot of people are taking meds for ills/medical conditions/ maladies/diseases that, not so long ago, were unrecognized as diseases requiring extensive, expensive and sometimes risky medical treatments. Examples include gastroesophageal reflux disease (25 million), seasonal allergic rhinitis (36 million), chronic dry eye (32 million) and restless leg syndrome (16 million). (Steve Wiegand and Dorsey Griffith, "In World of Drug Ads, There's A Pill for Every Ill," June 27, 2005.) Don't let Congress or anyone else medicalize your

31

health. Don't take any pills you are not certain you really need.

These are real problems, particularly reflux and dry eye, but not all require prescription medications for life and other extensive treatments. Sometimes, over-the-counter remedies serve nicely. Sometimes, unfortunately, extensive, expensive and sometimes risky medical treatments ARE in order—nothing less will bring relief or address the problem. Every senior should have a regular review of medications by a primary physician, during which all medications owned or taken since the last visit would be assessed. Perhaps this is the norm, but I kind of doubt it. Make it the norm for you as part of the preventive element of your AUI wellness program.

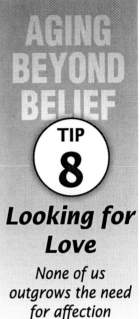

AGING
BEYOND
BELIEF

TIP

8

Looking for Love

None of us outgrows the need for affection

*A*s Waylon Jennings might express it, keep on searching their eyes, looking for traces of what you're dreaming of. In *The Beggars Opera*, John Gay wrote, "Youth's the season made for joys, Love is then our duty." Though well past that duty stage (the kids are grown, they have their own families, etc.), how about some loving affections, on an optional basis? After all, some of the things we do, though we are not compelled, often comprise life's sweetest pleasures.

In an interview at SeekWellness.com with Dr. Sol Gordon, the highly regarded educator, sex expert and author of "How Can You Tell If You're Really In Love" (*Adams Media*, Holbrook, MA., 2001) and many other books, I asked about looking for love, later in life. Sol advised that romance was good at any time in life, and noted that the ingredients of a successful relationship are a sense of humor, the wisdom to overlook a lot of stuff and respect for each other. Sol noted that many who start off "madly in love" end up just mad, so go easily on the "madly in love" part. The latter encourages jealousy that, though equated with love, is always destructive.

In the later stages of our voyage of discovery and self-development, we are most likely to have come closest to being the best person we can be—so we are ripe for love. Sol advises that couples focus on meaning and purpose, and do good deeds, without expectations of returns. Sol calls the latter "doing Mitzvahs," a rich part of the Jewish tradition.

I also asked Sol to identify the major roadblocks to love and intimacy. He mentioned unreal expectations of what love can do and suggested a question to ask yourself before committing to another, "In this person's presence, do I love myself more?" This Sol considers more important than hot sex and good times, as is having mental orgasms with each other rather than just the other kind, though both are nice. I asked Sol if he knew of any conflict-free relationships. He cited a Woody Allen movie (Annie Hall) wherein Woody's character goes up to a happy-looking couple and asks them their secret. The woman answers, "I'm very shallow and empty and I have no ideas and nothing interesting to say." Her man says, "And I'm exactly the same way." There you have one idea of what a conflict-free relationship might look like. But, probably not the kind that would be right for you. Be yourself, take chances and let the object of your socially-acceptable and other desires know what you're thinking. It's the best way to get what you want, some of the time.

*R*ecently, one of my best friends died. He was 83 and for a while had been the oldest person (at 77) to finish the Hawaiian Ironman Triathlon (since 2006, the record is age 80). More important, he was cheerful, optimistic and an inspiration to those who knew him, young and old, and to a great many others who had read or heard about him without having had the good fortune to appreciate him personally. Like Jim Ward, you too are a role model, whether you want to be or not. Inspire someone, as Jim inspired me, in your own fashion, by doing what you enjoy—with panache and grace in positive, optimistic ways.

The Right Perspective

Perspective is nearly everything, so set the standard and show the way

One of Jim's role-model strengths, and he had many, was his tendency to urge perspective. Most things are not such a big deal, IF viewed from a functional perspective. Jim had three favorite quotes, beginning with this one from Charlie Brown (Charles Schulz): "I've developed a new philosophy ... I only dread one day at a time." The other two were: "Worrying is like a rocking chair, it gives you something to do, but it gets you nowhere" (Glenn Turner) and "If you treat every situation as a life and death matter, you'll die a lot of times" (Dean Smith).

Stress is never in the event or circumstance, but the way we respond to it. As Samuel Clemens/Mark Twain wisely observed as Halley's comet neared for the second time in his life, "I am an old man and have known a great many troubles, but most of them never happened."

If you simply MUST worry about something, pick a threat far enough off that you might be dead before it happens. For example, worry about the fact that some astronomers think there's a two percent chance that a 350 meter-wide rock will collide with Earth on the 13th of April 2029. I'm kidding—don't fret about that, either.

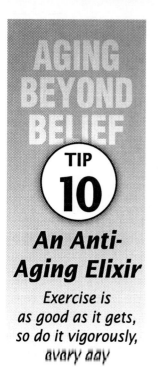

An Anti-Aging Elixir

Exercise is as good as it gets, so do it vigorously, every day

*B*eing fit is the closest thing we have to a panacea. Some older folks color their hair, wear a rug or plug their scalps, pop anti-aging pills/potions/and prescriptions and some even undergo cosmetic surgery to look younger. Save your money. Instead of these futilities, exercise. Regular exercise promotes physical vitality, which in turn is conducive to less dysfunctions and more psychological well-being. Both are great assets as the years accumulate. Exercise is vital at all stages of life but especially in the middle and later years. Exercise can make you feel better and enjoy life more, but doing enough of it is always a challenge. It is more of challenge after age 60, for example, than at age 30, at least physically. Yet, at 60 or older, regular exercise can improve all the life functions that it aided earlier in life and even mitigate the effects of some disabilities already experienced. It is also effective at improving mood and relieving depression. Most know that vigorous daily exercise is important but would rather not deal with it. However, middle age, if not treated with the mighty potion exercise, will invariably prove disastrous.

A classic Seinfeld episode dealt with aging. In the stand-up part of the show, Seinfeld talked about the relativity of aging. He discussed life today as much faster-paced than a few thousand years ago. "Today," Seinfeld noted, "life expectancy is around 76; back then, it was about 25! Put this in perspective. Among other things, it means that certain events we take for granted must have occurred much sooner for cavepersons. For instance, in those days, you got your driver's license at five, you were married at eight, your career peaked at twelve and social security kicked in at seventeen. If you encountered a person in later life, say, 22, you'd try to be polite—'Hey, you're really 22? Wow, you'd never know it. You look great for your age.'"

Recently, Garrison Keillor brought up aging in his monologue about "Lake Woebegon" on his popular radio show, *A Prairie Home Companion*. Keillor noted that time is like money. "It doesn't matter what you have SPENT, what matters is how much you've got left."

"Think of it this way," he said. "A man of 40 destined to live to 60 is actually older than a man of 50 who will live to 90. The 40 year-old thinks he's 10 years younger but actually he's 20 years older. In a way, then, you are only as young as you feel because the way you feel is an indication of how long you have left."

Keillor concluded by reflecting that getting older is a great adventure. "In a way, we're moving into a New Frontier, those of us growing older. We're all together in this wagon train. Some of us are farther ahead in the column than others." He stopped there but I'll add

the journey by speeding up your metabolism—with exercise done properly, every day. If you're only as old as you think, you will surely feel younger if you are fit and having fun and feeling good about how you look and what you are doing with the time that's left.

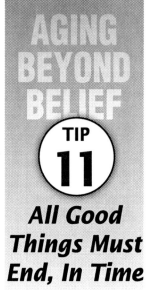

AGING BEYOND BELIEF

TIP 11

All Good Things Must End, In Time

Plan your own departure from this world

*N*obody likes to think about this, not even me, but I don't like to think about taxes, corruption, war profiteering, near-national bankruptcy, a losing foreign policy that endangers America, chronic incompetence, religious extremism, the shredding of the Constitution, gross hypocrisy, weakening of our defense, global warming, Mel Gibson and lots of things, but I try to stay informed and do what I must (i.e., pay taxes), anyway. Some things can be ignored, but many cannot, at least not without adverse consequences. Dying is in this latter category. Since we all have to ᴅᴏ ɪᴛ, ᴡʜy ɴᴏᴛ ᴛʀy ᴛᴏ ᴅᴏ ɪᴛ ᴄᴀʟᴍʟy, ɪꜰ ᴘᴏssɪʙʟᴇ? There are many reasons for planning an exit strategy while not in any immediate need of one. One reason is it's just not nice to wear out your welcome. Another is to avoid putting up with an extended, painful dying process that you would never allow a loved pet to endure. We should treat ourselves as well as we would treat Fido.

Of course, knowing when to hold and when to fold, under which circumstances, is a highly complicated issue. Formulas don't work very well. The best you can do is work out a few general principles, and communicate them to family, friends and a good lawyer. When the time comes to pull the proverbial plug, someone will know your wishes and have the decency to do what you would desire be done. Who should be responsible for making such a call, assuming you can't for one reason or another?

To boost your motivation to be in charge of this end-of-life choice, do a worst-case scenario—recall the infamous political grandstanding that accompanied the prolonged dying process of Terri Schiavo in Florida. Would you want to spend a decade or more in "a persistent vegetative state"—and be diagnosed by videotape by a politician quack doctor? Let me guess—not likely.

Check out the hospice movement. Also, peruse Internet resources to learn about such things as "The Hedonistic Imperative," the ingredients of a "Brompton Cocktail" and other pain relievers and end-of-life personal responsibility options. The idea is to spare family and friends the miseries and expenses of a drawn out decline. Unlike nearly all wellness matters, this subject is not a fun topic, but it is an important part of living to a not-so-bitter end.

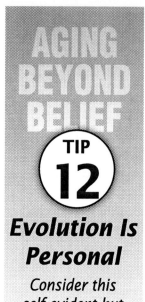

Evolution Is Personal

Consider this self-evident but disagreeable axiom— you can't be a kid forever

Everybody knows this at one level, but many unconscious desires, hopes and particularly frustrations occur when the reality of it is not accepted at the deepest, unconscious level. Getting old is not as good as being young in many ways, but it's life. Accept unavoidable facts as cheerfully as possible.

Two systems of concern are bones and muscles. In time, bones become less dense and lose mass and minerals. (This, of course, weakens the bones and makes them vulnerable to fracture.) Muscles also lose mass and strength, in part due to less water in the tendons and ligaments, leading to added stiffness. The cardiovascular system is affected because the size of the heart increases a little, as does blood pressure. More important, your maximal heart and heart recovery rates diminish. An ambitious fitness routine delays all this substantially, as Jack La Lanne (92) and others who live healthfully have demonstrated.

Unlike your bones and muscles, the decline of other body parts or systems with advancing age are less responsive to vigorous wellness lifestyle practices. That is to say, these systems are going to deteriorate whether you stand on your head, run marathons, eat a perfect diet (whatever that is) and do absolutely everything as well as it can be done. These systems include:

- Hearing—the cells of your inner ears are damaged by normal wear and tear of sounds over time. The auditory canal walls become thinner, eardrums thicken and it becomes more difficult to hear higher frequencies.

- Brainpower—The number of brain cells (neurons) diminish with age, though the number of connections between cells increase in some areas of the brain.

- Kidneys—The size of your kidneys and bladder capacity are reduced. The kidneys become less efficient at removing wastes from the blood.

- Reproduction—Men produce fewer sperm and suffer loss of testosterone; women produce less estrogen, progesterone and testosterone, for starters.

- Eyesight—There are losses in ability to produce tears, the retina gets thinner and the lens yellows. Almost everyone over forty learns the meaning of the word "presbyopia," a visual condition in which loss of elasticity of the lens of the eye causes defective accommodation and inability to focus sharply for near vision.

- Skin—You really do become "thin skinned," or at least your skin thins even if you don't become quick to take offense. Also, your sweat and oil (sebaceous) glands are less active and skin moisture decreases.

- Nails—Grow half as fast as they used to. Who cares? I suppose some women do, but of all the inevitable changes, this is one I won't mind in the slightest.

Of course, you never know, there may be extraordinary advances in the years to come. All you have to do is live long enough in order to benefit. However, be careful—some advances might never come to pass, in which case you could find yourself hanging around, waiting forever.

Many advances are on the horizon, it seems. Scientists just might develop impressive new memory-boosting strategies and life extension techniques. How? The possibilities are limitless. Maybe the key will be found in estrogen or testosterone. Maybe proteins of some kind or stem cells or gene therapies will be used to solve neurological problems associated with aging that will preserve cognitive function, prevent or cure Alzheimer's, asthma, AIDS, infectious diseases—and aging itself. Maybe, but probably not in time to work for you. The best strategy is to AUI of a wellness lifestyle.

The bottom line, if there is such a thing applied to aging, is how well and how long can you live? If you could discover how long, would you even WANT to know? No worries, since there IS no way of knowing, despite the compulsion of some futurists to make predictions.

On the other hand, we can greatly affect the quality of our lives. Life quality is very much subject to lifestyle actions, even if the ratio between birth and death will always be one to one. But clearly, old isn't what it used to be. By AUI of a wellness lifestyle, you can remain younger in important ways as long as possible. You will have to settle for that. It's the best a wellness lifestyle can provide, and it's worth a lot. Therefore, live well and enjoy each day.

*G*ive your grandchildren something special to complement your love, inheritance and good company—nurture their sense of wonder and respect for nature, science and reason.

If your grandson or granddaughter asks, "What's the upside to aging, grandma?" (or grandpa, as the case may be), resist the temptation to say, "Child, it's about becoming more attractive to the opposite sex, being athletically stronger and faster and quite funny and wealthy, too." But not for long. After a suitable pause during which time you are pretending to be thinking about the question, go ahead and say just that. Or words to similar effect. Your grandchild, if older than five, will crack up and be reinforced in her/his early mastery of an important lesson: Adults are a lot of fun, but their opinions, ideas, beliefs and worldviews are best taken with large doses of salt grains.

The Gift of Reason

Give your grandchildren a sense of wonder and respect for nature, science, and reason

There is a great deal of utter nonsense loose in the world, including a vast range of superstitions; "deceptive advertising" (excuse the redundancy), rumor, misinformation and myriad other forms of cognition gone astray. Such has always been the case, but the situation is even worse today. In some ways, this should not surprise—there are more people around in our time (about six billion) and the information age distributes nonsense as rapidly as other data. Yes, this is an era of unprecedented knowledge about the natural world, but a vast majority of the populace has not been keeping pace with or even paying attention to the extraordinary gains in the physical, natural and social sciences.

Your assignment, if you choose to accept it, is to become an agent of reason for your grandchildren. Yes, of course you might play the same role for your own children, friends and everyone else in your modest circle of influence. However, this tip is focused on urging you to consider the idea of passing along a unique, life-long gift to your grandchildren, a special legacy of "mental modeling" over time.

I have no idea HOW you might carry out this tip! You may not even have grandchildren and if you do, they may be too young to influence and so on. If this is the case, try to relate this tip to other people in your sphere of influence, if the promotion of reason strikes you as important and interesting. How could it not?

In general terms, the way to approach this role is to offer, in your own style and fashion, a good-natured presence for reason and the wonders of nature. Communicate in varied ways the idea that all things are best understood, or at least studied, through free inquiry.

If you agree that there is merit in this tip, here are perspectives to consider. Please take account of such views in communications with the grandkids, and everyone else.

- Our society is powered by science and technology. Both are best understood with a philosophy based upon a joy in discovery, not a philosophy steeped in the defense of dogmatisms, creeds or ideologies.

- Fantasies and myths entertain and comfort. Before the age of reason, it may not be ruinous to go along with quaint cultural traditions that are probably harmless if silly and irrational, such as belief in Santa Claus, the Easter Bunny and the Tooth Fairy. However, the promotion of these and similar myths to a child who has reached grade school may not be the best preparation for future adults who will need to know about the world as it really is.

- We can't all be Carl Sagans, Stephen Jay Goulds, Paul Kurtzs, Isaac Asimovs, Richard Dawkins', Bill Nyes or other brilliant and influential scientists, but we can make a difference in modest ways. Explore with the grandkids and others the discoveries available in the works of science popularizers.

- An understanding can grow as much from questions as from answers. You could ask a teen for examples of how our culture propagates baloney. This could lead to a fun conversation about what is the nature of pseudoscience and superstition, and how are these phenomena different from science? How can you not provoke a great discussion with such a suggested agenda? No need to convince anyone of anything. You want people to think, not consent. A provocative discussion represents another occasion to arouse curiosities that invite further mulling, in time. This role is about thinking, not resolutions.

- Avoid polarization. Modeling a respect for reason as a preferred way to make decisions does not include an "Us vs. Them" shortcut approach in thinking. Resist temptations to condescend, belittle or signal arrogance, even toward those who embrace and even advocate what seem to be irrational beliefs. Many smart people have been acculturated to be credulous—it is more common that you might realize. We all have our weaknesses and frailties. An important trait to model for others is that of compassion—and tolerance, respect and kindness.

- Encourage young minds (and old ones, too) to try to confirm alleged facts and, if a given topic is of special interest and warrants more time and energy, to seek out knowledgeable proponents of all points of view.

- Find ways to talk about and give examples of sound thinking regarding current events. Let the grandkids know about logical and rhetorical fallacies. These are too numerous to list and describe here, but you will want to familiarize yourself with at least the following: Arguments from authority that rely on a single hypothesis to explain something, arguments that lack quantification, arguments that are missing chains in a line of an argument, or propositions that can't be tested or falsified.

And this is just the start of things to consider or, in your case, to introduce to the grandkids and/or others in your circle of influence.

Other important ideas to convey include issues surrounding the influence of controls and multiple variables and fallacies of logic and rhetoric. Among the most prevalent are personal attacks (ad hominem), reliance on authority to persuade (i.e., Grand Poobah assertions called "arguments from authority") and arguments from adverse consequences (e.g., "If such and such were not so, well then, all hell would break loose").

Are you thinking that's the end of it? Can it get more irrational than that? Yes, I'm just warming up. There is so much more to warn against if you want to help the grandchildren think better than most of us who have come before them. Obviously, it's a good idea to set modest expectations in managing this tip of being a role model for promoting reason.

Think of the heralded superstar advocates for reason and science that I have already mentioned above—Sagan, Gould, Kurtz, Asimov, Dawkins and Nye. They wrote books, made films, gave countless lectures, had TV shows, wrote influential articles and so on. Who can match that—and yet they have not changed society all that much, it would appear. Despite their prodigious efforts, are we not still awash in pseudoscience, ignorance, irrationality and other dysfunctional states? If their extraordinary, watershed contributions and those of thousands of others doing similar good work in promoting science and reason have not turned the tide, what chance do you have? If that's what you are thinking, not to worry. You must not expect too much from your efforts. Just a little influence on a life or two, especially the lives of little relatives, perhaps, who are of special interest and concern. Do this and you will have impact aplenty—with a bit of personal satisfaction as your reward.

No, I have not overlooked such common logical fallacies as appeal to ignorance, special pleading, straw man, slippery slope, begging the question, observational selection (or enumeration of favorable circumstances), what Francis Bacon described as "counting the hits and forgetting the misses." In addition, there are additional fallacies common in our public life, such as people using statistics of small numbers, misunderstanding of the nature of statistics, inconsistency in the use of data, using non sequiturs and arguments that are "post hoc, ergo propter hoc" and so on. Think of the possibilities for the influence you can have with this tip. The battles to pick, the targets to attend are so incredibly numerous and deserving of demolition. A few others are known as fallacies of suppressed evidence, weasel words, meaningless questions, excluded middle (the false dichotomy) and so on. The list is quite daunting, which reinforces the importance of the grandparent role I have suggested. There is a treasure trove of additional information available to wonder-promoting grandparents at countless websites, one of my favorites being www.fallacyfiles.org. This site lists many other excellent sources.

As Carl Sagan, author of the famous "baloney detection kit" observed, the forces of irrationality have a huge arsenal of deception at their disposal. Almost anything can be misused, taken out of context and otherwise manipulated to deceive and exploit—and such things are done daily on a massive scale.

For these reasons, I hope you will find the tip about giving grandchildren something special to complement your love, inheritance and good company to be an appealing and doable idea. What better gift than to nurture another's sense of wonder and respect for nature, science and reason. I would think this would be right up there with the dazzling range of other benefits of your presence in their lives.

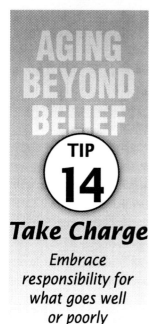

AGING BEYOND BELIEF

TIP 14

Take Charge

Embrace responsibility for what goes well or poorly

Make the best of whatever happens, whether positive or negative. Embracing responsibility will serve you better than playing the blame game, making excuses, whining and whimpering, shifting accountability or suing somebody. In this fashion, you might be able to minimize your need for medical services. Doctors, drugs, and the medical system can be invaluable, when used appropriately and truly needed. However, the determinant of health you most control is lifestyle—the choices either positive (e.g., exercising regularly) or negative (e.g., smoking) that you make, for better or worse, over time. The other key factors—genetics, environment and the medical system, are either set in place (genetics) or difficult to change (environmental factors) in the near term.

However much I tout the potency of a strong sense of personal responsibility, human decency and common sense it's imperative that I acknowledge a tragic reality, namely, some people are just dealt a bad hand. The older you get, the more instances you can cite of family members, friends, associates and/or others who took very good care of themselves with exemplary lifestyles, but were felled anyway, by any number of fatal diseases. I'll refrain from dwelling upon the mournful fact about inequities as part of the human experience, but it's worth remembering nonetheless.

Do you still have that "youthful glow and step?" No matter—most of us can do nicely without the glow and step of youth. There are other attractions, such as having fun doing things outrageous, exciting, almost illegal and often at odds with cultural norms. No, I'm not going to suggest you take ecstasy, smoke pot, attend rave concerts, dress ridiculously or have premature ejaculations, although one or more of these may have some attractions.

Time travel is still off a bit in the future, so you have to improvise to move back in time, in a functional sense. There are no guaranteed methods for doing this, but there are a few mini-tips related to responsibility that can, for a while, make you feel younger.

1. Get ridiculously fit. Select an activity that requires serious training and set a goal that will take at least three months to achieve. This will make you feel dramatically younger—guaranteed.

2. Work on your sense of humor. Decide that you will double the number of "light" moments you experience daily. This will entail going out of your way to pursue humor in ways that otherwise might not have been attempted. Be imaginative, be bold and be a little outrageous in your quest.

3. Reconnect with someone from high school or college whom you have not heard from for at least a decade! This person may or may not have been a lover or object of fantasies or other desires in earlier times. Just pick someone with whom the quest for a reunion by phone, letter or, best of all, in person, will prove a bit exciting. Even if the actual reconnection is nothing special, getting there will have been fun.

4. Go back to college. Do this even if you never went to college! Take a course, preferably on an audit basis (cheaper), or just crash a single class. If you are old enough, they will assume you are a distinguished professor and will be honored by your presence. The other possibility is they will think you a bit daft, in which case they'll leave you alone. Pick a subject area that interests you and don't be shy about asking tough questions that get to the heart of the matter. Why? Because even if you're feeling youthful, you don't have forever to get to the bottom of things.

5. Have a guilt-free orgasm in a matter a little out of the ordinary. Be bold and daring. Go beyond your boundaries now and

then. These things are not a violation of sensible morality, nor are they illegal, except in Alabama.

6. Do something really wacky, but harmless. Come to the dinner table dressed as an ape or something (great costumes can be rented very cheaply in every city in the US and Canada—and the costume shops are a lot of fun to peruse.)

7. Visit a nudist resort, walk or jog naked in the woods, dance in the altogether with a friend, skinny-dip in a lake or do something fun without clothes on. This will really make you feel younger and, unlike my first tip, does not require months of preparation or heavy breathing.

Some of these things might not turn out so well. If that proves to be the case, well, remember the title of this tip—be responsible for what goes well or poorly. That is, don't blame me!

Allow for the possibility that you could be around a very long time, maybe even to age 100. Act accordingly. The chances are better than you probably think. There are no less than 50,000 American centenarians. Any idea what the number was a century ago? Nearly none! The forecast for 2050, a date just around the corner more or less, is for 800,000 to one million Americans 100 or more.

What are the factors that could boost your lifespan, besides your own efforts at staying fit, eating well, having fun and so on? A partial list might include fancy, whiz bang genetically engineered hormones, advances in genomics, biotechnology, nanotechnology and so on that interact positively with diet, metabolism, genetics, toxins and the rest. There may be new ways to strengthen your immune system, rejuvenate your tissues and organs and slow the aging process on a cellular level.

Some crackpot might offer a diet plan that, contrary to most if not all diet plans for the past century or so, works! Not likely, but it's possible, I suppose. Maybe it will feature something not tried before that turns out to be surprisingly effective, like alkaline water mixed with lemons and formaldehyde. (I'm kidding—don't try this at home.)

Well, I suppose IF you can just hold on long enough, you can last almost forever. But, what a huge IF! I could fly, too, IF only I had wings and a more aerodynamic skull.

Of course, even if every disease known to man were eradicated, living forever might be tricky given the continued existence of wars, especially of the thermonuclear kind, the growth of murderous religious fanaticism and, of course, the huge popularity of ghastly lifestyle choices made by the masses. In short, the case for longevity AND vitality much beyond the century mark is somewhere between ludicrous and comical.

You are NOT going to live forever. Not even close. However, that's no reason to eschew the bright side of life and be as well as possible, for as long as you do hold on. Bottom line: Don't dwell on longevity; instead, make the most of the present. "Millions long for immortality who do not know what to do with themselves on a rainy Sunday afternoon." (Susan Ertz, *Anger in the Sky*, 1943.) Steven Wright said, "I intend to live forever; so far, so good."

*T*his is because you may not last a long time, especially if you are "normal" (i.e., overweight and underfit). Recall this immortal advice from Erma Bombeck: "Seize the moment. Remember all those women on the Titanic who waved off the dessert cart."

While the American lifespan is much better now than in 1900 (77.3 years versus 47.3 years), don't expect this trend line to continue. Many experts in life expectancy believe positive trend lines do not take account of the disastrous effects of rampant obesity. So, to paraphrase an immortal line, "Ask not how long can I live; ask how well can I live?" This is where play comes into the picture.

TIP
16

Have Fun, Stay Busy

Enjoy as much dessert (play) as possible, without delays

Play will give you energy boosts while reducing boredom and burnout. Broaden your thinking about the nature of play. Think of play as being in nature, communing with the land, fauna and wildlife, as well as participating in sporting events. All are forms of play. You might derive great pleasure from hiking in wilderness areas or photographing wildlife in the natural world. No need to create a hierarchy of play with higher, dignified, socially approved and ennobling forms at one end and lowlife forms (e.g., mud wrestling) at another—all forms are useful, provided nobody gets hurt and the horses are not frightened.

Some of my favorite (anonymous) quotes deal with play, particularly when exercise and eating dessert are included as elements of such.

- Fifty years ago people finished a day's work and needed rest. Today they finish and need exercise.

- If you are going to try cross-country skiing, start with a small country.

- I'm in shape—round is a shape, isn't it?

- Aerobics defined: A series of strenuous exercises which help convert fats, sugars, and starch into aches, pains and cramps.

- No diet will remove all the fat from your body because the brain is entirely fat. Without a brain, you might look good, but all you could do is run for public office. (Actually, this one is not anonymous—it's been attributed to George Bernard Shaw.)

Well, the lessons seem clear enough: play will do you a world of good. Play all the days of your life, until you die when, for the first time in life, it won't matter anymore.

I shared the podium at a wellness conference in West Virginia around 1989 with then 89-year old Maggie Kuhn (1905-1995), founder of the Gray Panthers organization. Maggie joked about the outrageous things she could say and do because of her advanced age. This outrageousness aided in the growth of the Gray Panthers as an intergenerational organization that continues to this day. Take advantage of the added freedom to ignore norms and customs that inhibit your best self. Be the "wild and crazy kind of guy" (or gal) Steve Martin used to talk about. John Stuart Mill advised as much when he wrote, "The amount of eccentricity in a society has generally been proportional to the amount of genius, mental vigor and moral courage it contained. That so few dare to be eccentric marks the chief danger of the time." (*On Liberty*, 1859.)

Speak Up, Make a Fuss

Don't be shy— you can get away with a lot the older you are

One way to overcome a lingering reticence to shake things up is to become more outspoken. Consider the fact that you have many more years of experience than most people—why not give others the benefit of your accumulated knowledge and wisdom? Start pontificating, like a philosopher, about your lifestyle (with wellness anecdotes, hopefully) and your opinions on politics, sex and religion. Philosophy is, after all, just the love and pursuit of wisdom by intellectual means and moral self-discipline, something you know plenty about. It entails an investigation of causes and laws underlying reality. That's exactly what you have been doing in seeking excellence in body and mind.

To balance this bright wit with some dim wit, here is one of the single most muddled passages I ever encountered, from a holistic eccentric with a big following, namely Deepak Chopra: "The truth is, I'm here, but I am also everywhere else; that you're there, but you're also here, because here is there and there is everywhere and, of course, everywhere is nowhere, specifically." (From a Chopra audiotape entitled *Escaping The Prison of the Intellect*.) My sense from pondering the above statement is that the guru made good his escape.

Deepak's assault on lucidity was put in perspective by Jack Raso, editor of *Nutrition Forum* (July/August, 1994, page 42), who noted: "I, for one, would think twice before asking Chopra for directions."

Be a bit eccentric and go against the norms, if it helps you to be your best and overcome at least a few obstacles to a healthy and satisfying lifestyle. Seek a healthier lifestyle, look for health in all the right places and make disciplined choices. Enjoy the process, keep learning and tell everyone else what you have discovered at every opportunity.

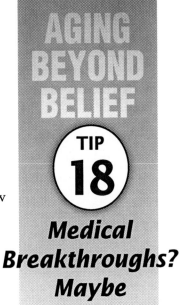

TIP
18

Medical Breakthroughs? Maybe

Curb your enthusiasm —the latest study findings are nothing to get excited about

*S*ensationalism sells newspapers but does not contribute a lot to what you need to know about good nutrition. Be cautious, even skeptical, of news reports about diet research. If researchers themselves claim a breakthrough of some kind, which reputable scientists rarely do (e.g., "Our new longitudinal study suggests that high fat, alcohol-rich diets boost brain power"), don't get your hopes up. Wait for corroboration from additional studies before assuming that any claims, especially big ones, have merit.

Do you ever wonder why so many people are still confused about the nature of a healthy diet? For that matter, why am I still confused about the nature of a healthy diet, not to mention the surest path to unbounded happiness, the meaning of life and unbounded fame and riches? Here's my theory. I think it explains all these matters regarding the absence of certainty.

It's because certainty is not an option! There is little certainty available about anything. Reporters and others in the media world do not favor nuanced headlines, so they underplay uncertainty, even when they appreciate the fact of it. Sweeping statements that ignore limitations are the best way for them to do business, under current conditions. However, no need for you to be fooled. Just be suspicious of breakthroughs about diet and other claims that contradict established scientific standards.

The good news is that sound and reliable evidence regarding good diet is extensive. Such guides as moderate your intake of certain types of fats (saturated, trans, partially hydrogenated), salt and sugar in favor of more whole grains, fruit and vegetables are well-supported by science. Good information about nutrition is not hard to find.

One of my favorite resources is the UC Berkeley "Wellness Letter," www.wellnessletter.com; another is The Center for Science in the Public Interest (CSPI), www.cspinet.org

So, curb your enthusiasm for the latest studies, eat less and move more. Also, get on with your unique quest for the surest path to unbounded happiness, the meaning of life and great fame and riches.

*F*or long life, your level of education is more influential than health insurance, wealth, race, gender, location, support system—even how much sex you enjoy (or suffer). That's a fact, based upon research at the National Institute on Aging and many other studies over the years. Of course, it's not known why higher levels of education correlate with longer life, but it does. So, consider going back to college, joining a fraternity or sorority and having a good time, as in the good old days gone by.

Learning— A Key to Longevity

Get more education, whatever your age

OK, I'm not really advocating you go to that extreme, though it might be fun. The point is this: Keep learning new stuff, even if it's not really a factor in lasting longer. It's just a better way to be alive.

Scientists speculate why more education equates with longevity. Can you guess their best guesses? Basically, it comes to this: The more educated you are, the less likely you were to have smoked and done other self-destructive things over the course of your life—and more likely to have had better jobs and more control over your work life.

Also, less healthy kids or those from poorer families may have been less able to sustain extensive schooling, meaning education was really a proxy for favored family economics. Further, wealthier families who supported their children for extended educations also provided better nutrition. The latter could be the key factor, not education (which would be a symptom or corollary of greater wealth).

When these and other factors are thoroughly scrutinized, it appears that:

- Cohesive social networks are crucial. Such ties have long been associated with greater longevity.

- Poorly educated people are less inclined to plan for the future and delay gratification. This partly explains why high-risk behaviors are much greater within this class.

- Wealth buys health, to some degree (access to the best medical care, drugs and housing, etc.)—higher education is, naturally, associated with increased wealth.

It seems the cliché "living in the moment" or for today may not always be such a good thing. One expert on longevity studies observed, "It's the worst thing for your health. Most of adherence (to wise health habits) is unpleasant. You have to be willing to do something that is not pleasant now and you have to stay with it and think about the future." (Quoted in an article by Gina Kolata, "A Surprising Secret to a Long Life: Stay in School," *New York Times*, January 3, 2007.)

There are still many ways to stimulate your brain in order to remain as sharp as possible late in life. In the last year or so, there has been a surge in products and programs specifically designed as fitness routines for your hippocampus, temporal lobe and brain parts. An interesting summary of these innovations appeared at the end of last year in an article by Pam Belluck in the *New York Times* entitled, "As Minds Age, What's Next? Brain Calisthenics?" (December 27, 2006). Could these tools enable a cognitive fountain of youth of sorts? With few downside risks in evidence, it seems worth a try. Of course, none of the tools are a sure thing in all cases, but aging centers find sufficient promise in this area to invest in "brain gyms" that promote mental exercise routines. The goals are to aid memory, reasoning abilities and/or processing speed—and success at any one of these targeted outcomes would make such initiatives well worth the time, cost and effort. The American Society on Aging, the AARE the Alzheimer's Association, two major health insurers (MetLife and Humana) and a few corporations (e.g., Nintendo, Apple Computer and Lockheed Martin) are pushing brain health. Web sites like www.HappyNeuron. com (cranial calisthenics) and www.MyBrainTrainer.com) have been established to focus on brain training for seniors.

In the Times article noted, the chief of health care and aging studies at the federal Centers for Disease Control and Prevention(which is charged by Congress to study brain health enhancements) is quoted as follows: "What's good for your heart's probably good for your head." This is the key, in my view. If you are exercising vigorously on a daily basis and eating well, you are automatically looking after your brain, as well. It makes sense to go the next step, which is to experiment with varied mind training games and routines that show promise—of psychological if not actual cognitive benefits.

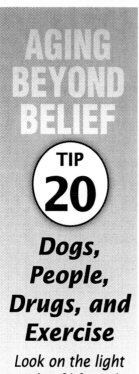

AGING BEYOND BELIEF

TIP 20

Dogs, People, Drugs, and Exercise

Look on the light side of life and aging ... learn a new trick or two

What can you do but laugh at some human foibles? It turns out that sedentary people are a bad influence on their dogs, so much so that the FDA recently approved a prescription medication for treating canine obesity. What are we coming to? We live in a mad world. I got a subscription for dogs for the FDA to consider—exercise. Rumor has it that it works for pudgy people, too. (See "New Diet Drug Is Approved for Pudgy Dogs, New York Times, January 6, 2007.)

Did you know that five percent of dogs in this country are estimated to be overweight, according to vets who track this sort of thing? That comes to four million tubby mutts. The head of Pfizer, which sells the drug ("Slentrol") for a couple bucks per daily dosage, claimed (in the above noted New York Times article) that it would help owners unable unwilling or unable to cut back on treats given to their pets. A pity, since obesity, as in their masters, is associated with doggie cardiovascular problems, diabetes, torn ligaments, elbow sores, hip and back problems and arthritis. (Maybe sore elbows are not the biggest worry for obese humans.) As with humans, exercise is vastly more effective, but much more labor intensive (time, sweat and heaving breathing required) than taking drugs.

If you are not already an athletic person, please give yourself and, if you have one, your dog a good dose of daily exercise. Think of it as a new trick. Of course, dogs don't usually have to be persuaded or coerced to exercise—a Frisbee or passing car can set them into an aerobic frenzy that would put a champion athlete to shame. But, they need humans to give them such opportunities if not allowed to roam about on their own. The latest study shows that doggie workouts, along with a diet fortified with vitamins, fruits and vegetables, helps old dogs learn new tricks. (I'm reminded of a "Far Side" cartoon by Gary Larson. A dog is shown paused on a high wire overlooking a circus crowd, looking down while holding a balance beam. The caption reads: "High above the hushed crowd, Rex tried to remain focused. Still, he couldn't shake one nagging thought: He was an old dog, and this was a new trick.")

Actually, exercise has been shown to HELP old dogs learn new tricks. Why not humans, too? Who wouldn't like to learn a new trick or two?

Dogs are similar to humans in dietary needs (and the way they digest food) and, like us, experience memory and learning problems with age. A study showed an antioxidant diet and lots of cognitive stimulation made old dogs better at thinking, in other words, capable of new tricks (to use doggie imagery).

Those of us getting older (i.e., everyone) should consider boosting diets with lots of tomatoes, carrot granules, citrus pulp, spinach and supplements while getting extra exercise and play. These factors did wonders for Rex and his mates under controlled conditions at the Institute of Aging —I'm sure the regimen will help you, too.

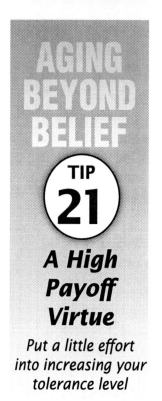

AGING BEYOND BELIEF

TIP

21

A High Payoff Virtue

Put a little effort into increasing your tolerance level

One way to stay happier is by reducing opportunities for unhappiness. Over time, by a determination not to sweat the little stuff and a mindset that it's all ultimately little stuff, you can fashion an ironclad suit of armor against all manner of vexations. There is no gain in allowing yourself to be disturbed by religions, lifestyles, appearances and opinions at variance with your own. Block the annoyances of daily life and you will suffer fewer mini-states of unhappiness, if any at all. (I need to work on this one in order not to become less happy every time I see or hear certain Republican politicians.) Live your own life and let others do the same. They are going to, anyway. People are too hard to reform.

Let's look at the basics for just a moment. Tolerance is a noun meaning "sympathy or indulgence for beliefs or practices differing from or conflicting with one's own" (Merriam-Webster). It is a vital ingredient for successful democracies. The rights of everyone, especially those in a minority, are much safer in a tolerant culture populated by people sympathetic to or indulgent toward divergent beliefs and practices. Tolerance surely warrants a high ranking on any list of valuable wellness traits. An epiphany is a "sudden manifestation or perception of the essential nature or meaning of something." To have an epiphany, say about tolerance, is to experience "an intuitive grasp of reality simple and striking, an illuminating discovery, a revealing scene or moment."

My epiphany is that tolerance, like a physically fit body, is something you have to work on and cultivate, day in and day out. Like a high performance body, it is not easy to achieve and even harder to maintain. If fitness and tolerance were easy, everyone would be fit and tolerant—and you know that isn't the case.

One of my favorite workouts for developing a somewhat better proficiency at tolerance is to observe fundamentalist religious zealots on any given day—and notice whether I was able to resist a sense of dismay, anger or revulsion. Also, I note whether I could resist the temptation to seek an Australian visa.

In any event, the epiphany I mentioned earlier about how I need to practice tolerance was reinforced the other day (April 24, 2004) reading an article by Nicholas D. Kristof in the *New Yorlk Times* entitled, "Hug an Evangelical." THAT, I knew, would not be easy. Even Kristof acknowledged that it's no cakewalk for him, either. Among Kristof's obstacles to hugging an evangelical are such vexations as:

- Strident, allegedly bible-based discrimination against gays and lesbians ("Conservative Christians should show a tad more divine love for homosexuals."). I'm neither, but I can't see any reason to discriminate against them—or anyone else. Except religious extremists, but as I noted, I'm working on that. That's why I wrote this tip—primarily for me!

- A propensity by some conservative Christians to be a tad judgmental (in other words, they are "all too quick to sentence outsiders to hell").

- Continuous efforts by these Christian "hypocritical blowhards" to impose their symbols on society, including Ten Commandment plaques, the "under God" phrase in civic rituals and on coins, restrictive sexual mores in laws and creationism rather than science in classrooms public and private.

The rest of us, Kristof suggests, should work on our tolerance by being more respectful and less contemptuous of evangelicals. Hmmmm. Working on it.

It's worth noting that tolerance should not be equated or confused with the surrender of treasured elements of free speech. The latter occurs with campus speech codes under the restrictions of political correctness. Let's protect our rights to engage in somewhat constructive (and irreverent) criticism. While we're at it, let's not give away our freedoms to offer opinions that some may not appreciate, as well as the option to attempt humor that may or may not amuse. And one more thing—to retain the right to express wonder at human follies—especially those that threaten our constitutional (if not "God-given") rights. The president insists freedom comes from "the Almighty." Maybe, but I tend to think freedom comes from the founders, via the Constitution, especially the Bill of Rights. However, getting back to the point of this tip, I can be tolerant of varied interpretations even as I wonder about how stingy the Almighty seems to have been distributing freedom across the world during the short span of human history. After all, as Kristof reminds us, even as we do our most strenuous of tolerance aerobics, "religion is much too important an influence on policy to be a taboo."

Consider this—the way to achieve true tolerance is the same approach essential to exceptional physical fitness or being invited to perform at Carnegie Hall —practice, practice, practice.

For one thing, the sacrifices might prove not helpful and the pleasures foregone might turn out to have had health benefits. (That's how I feel about not eating cashew nuts, though I'm thinking of switching to pistachios.) Excess in moderation, that's the ticket. Curiously, freedom from vices is NOT a characteristic of the longest of the long-lived. Many centarians turn out to be junk food junkies, most seem given to drink (in moderation) and a few, believe it or not, are couch potatoes. Frenchwoman Jeanne Calment, who at 122 was the oldest person before she gave up her title by dying, was a smoker! Go figure. Perhaps, if she had taken better care of herself, she would be alive and well still, and maybe even a perennial top finisher in her age group in local triathlons. Or, consider the recently departed Christian Mortensen of Marin County, CA, born August 16, 1882 in Denmark. A friend remarked, "He drank 20 glasses of water daily and he said his vice of smoking cigars helped him relax. He had a very good sense of humor. He liked to joke. He also was a very independent man." His death was reported in the local newspaper, the *Independent Journal*. Someone said, "He died peacefully in his sleep. The day before he said he felt great." I'm not sure who's the oldest now, but it's not me. However, as Parkinson once noted, "the future lies ahead," so I may yet become a contender.

Which reminds me of a conversation that took place recently amongst a group of retirees. They were talking about their ailments. One said, "My arms are so weak I can hardly hold this cup of coffee." Another added, "Yes, I know. My cataracts are so bad I can't even see my coffee." Someone else replied, "I can't turn my head because of the arthritis in my neck." A fourth chipped in, as all present nodded in agreement, "My blood pressure pills make me dizzy."

TIP

22

Living Longer Versus Living Well

Don't give up everything you enjoy in hopes of living a little longer

After someone else said, "I guess that's the price we pay for getting old," there was a moment of silence. Then, another remarked, cheerfully, "Well, it's really not all that bad—thank God we can all still drive!"

Whatever your age or condition, there is something to be cheerful about. Not everyone might find it cause for celebration, but you can, so don't miss a single opportunity to be grateful to the stars, or something, for anything you can be grateful about.

Stress management skills are an art form. No, they won't make you younger, nor will they alter the realities of unwanted changes. However, they will make a positive difference in the quality of your remaining days—or decades. Mastering stress will mitigate many challenges to your serenity and sense of meaning. Applying stress management principles will also buffer against the unsettling fact that the world is increasingly populated by people much younger than you are.

There are bright-side alternatives to cursing the darkness, joining a cult, dwelling in a state of semi or full-blown misery or retreating to the comforts of medications, TV or shuffleboard tournaments. On the other hand, maybe shuffleboard IS a bright side option—your choice.

Staying Centered and Balanced

Minimize negative stresses as much as possible

In America, life expectancy is very close to 78 years, but that fact does not carry with it any guarantees. Due to chance, genetics, environment and lifestyle factors, you may live much longer, or not so long. But don't count on setting records, like living to 120—the agreed upon limit for documented human survival. Consider that most who make it to 78 are not always elated about it. As the government sponsored project "Healthy People" reported, the final 11.7 years of life for most Americans are endured by at least one and often additional life-quality diminishing disabilities.

In a longevity context, consider the evolving consensus among researchers and scholars that successfully managing stress is the underrated key to a healthy, long life. On the other side, those who function day in and day out in a perpetual state of road rage (even when not driving!), subject their bodies to conditions that will do them in. This dysfunctional emotional state is as perilous as being a sedentary, overweight, junk food addict. Unfortunately, some folks combine the latter with high stress emotional states.

To improve the chances of extending your own lifespan AND reducing the likelihood of disabilities, four qualities, all accepted as the gold standard of longevity, are advised:

1. Manage your stress.

2. Become and remain fit.

3. Eat wisely in accord with the known science of needed nutrients.

4. Inherit good genes.

Three of these four are manageable, as are two other factors— personality and social life. The latter are important chiefly because of their influence on your capacity for stress management. Stress does more to age you than time, at least during the middle years, which I figure occur between 40 and 70.

Studies using non-human subjects demonstrate the important role of plentiful exercise and sound diet on critter longevity. In combination with human studies, consistent results have convinced researchers that stress is an underrated aging variable. All such studies, whether of rats, monkeys, nuns, British government workers or centenarians, support this finding. (See Living Better, Living Longer; Harvard Health Publications; National Vital Statistics Reports, Centers for Disease Control.)

Researchers are most interested in HOW unmanaged negative stress causes premature aging. However, speculations on why stress impacts longevity follow readily from an understanding of the basic fight/flight response. Current thinking about how stress, such as fear, anger, anxiety, worry and so on, leads to an early grave can be summarized as follows. When stress arises, the body responds automatically, the better to set you up to deal effectively with the stressor. Glucose goes to the muscles and there is an increase in heart and breathing rates, as well as blood pressure. Stress hormones are released that dull pain and sharpen senses. All this enables more oxygen to flow throughout the body. In case you catch a spear or something in the neck, not to worry too much—your blood vessels will have constricted while blood clotting has increased, both of which will slow the bleeding. At the same time, and this is really cool, processes not so important for the fight or flight option or full body alert are suppressed. These include digestion and immune functions—they can wait a while. Also, forget sexual arousal during action periods—the stress response eliminates the sex drive. Time for that later, if you survive.

In other words, the parts and systems of the body that you need for action are aroused, while the rest go on sleep mode. You need muscles to function at top speed, and rapid functioning of the heart, lungs and so on. Yet, you can't stay at war all the time—and sustain good health. In fact, this "Def-Com"-like red alert situation takes a terrible toll over time. Go on such alerts too often, as in many times daily if a stressed-out lifestyle kamikaze, and you are going to wear out—fast. Forget 120 years—you'll be lucky to live long enough to join AARP. As expressed by Tara-Parker Pope in the above-cited *Wall Street Journal* article, "... unremitting stress—in a person who can't shed it—leaves the stress response in the 'on' position. All those changes that protect you in a moment of crisis suddenly turn on you. Now you're just a person with unregulated blood sugar, high blood pressure, blood clots, a depressed sex drive and an immune system buckling under all the strain. It sounds a lot like getting old."

You know if you are a high stress person. It is not easy to change— very few lifestyle changes that matter are easy to reform. Yet, the stakes are so high, especially in older people for whom the stress response lasts longer. Thus, all efforts to chill out are worth the trouble, however difficult. Different approaches work for different people depending on many factors, but experiment with many techniques if you are one who experiences the stress response to excess.

The first line of resistance to the adverse consequences of the stress response is a healthy body. Start your "chill out" program by getting more sleep, exercise and emotional support. Then, develop coping skills. Develop strong social and family relationships and get connected—don't settle into a pattern wherein you are alone most of the time. Seek out a network of companions, friends and lovers—even a mate (though the reasons for the latter should extend beyond stress management!). Find ways to increase the control you have at work and home, your sense of security and your authority levels (for example, get a dog and lots of plants). Work on becoming happier and developing a delightful sense of humor. Laugh it up as much as you (and others) can bear! Adopt a positive outlook, even if you have to fake it. Eventually, it will get easier. Choose to be as optimistic as you can, even when it is not justified! Value and practice these and other personality traits known to diminish the stress response. The broad goal is adaptability to change and a willingness to experiment with new things. All these traits are linked to better aging—so start today by thinking of at least half a dozen ways you can minimize stress in your life.

*L*earn to wield these benign arts in order
to enrich your life and contribute to affable
community relations. Doing so will be much to
your advantage. Too often, we are disappointed
or offended by the absence of such qualities.
Etiquette, courtesy and good manners are three
closely related and complementary qualities.
Yet, each has its own meanings and applications.
All are vital to a smooth and enjoyable sense of
shared values and a supportive community.

TIP

24

Being Polite

*Use etiquette,
courtesy, and good
manners in an
artful manner for
your enjoyment, as
a service to others,
and because it's
good for you*

Judith Martin, best known as "Miss Manners,"
believes "freedom without rules doesn't work."
Edith Wharton, Henry James and legions of
pacesetters (or enforcers of established refined
sensibilities!) would surely concur. Similarly,
healthy lifestyles without due consideration
for the sensibilities of others does not work
so well, either, especially for purposes of harmonious, successful
relationships.

It's never too late in life to learn new refinements and add to your
panache and style. As George Eliot observed, "What do we live for
if not to make life less difficult for each other?" Well, I can think of
other reasons for living, but this is surely a good one to add to the
mix.

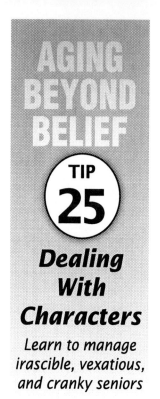

If you ARE an irascible, vexatious or cranky senior, change your ways, please! You might give other seniors a bad reputation!

There are three good reasons to develop this skill and put it into practice. One—they need help. Nobody is happy being a crank. Two –guiding such folks to lighten up will benefit everyone who otherwise is going to be stressed by their presence. Thus, you'll be performing a public service. Three—artfully managing a situation involving unreasonable people will prove enjoyable and satisfying. There is much mirth and devilish delight to be gained from doing so artfully and with panache. The famed philosopher, Mr. Anonymous, is rumored to have remarked, "It's hard to be religious when there are certain people who are never incinerated by bolts of lightning."

Turning them (the cranks) around with a bit of sleigh of tongue and response is less dramatic than lightening bolts, but you can never count on lightening bolts when you need them.

Of course, most seniors are so nice, so agreeable and so positive. Here is an example of a typical senior (!). It's almost surely apocryphal, but the syrupy, urban legend-like tale made its way around the Internet recently and it does connect with this tip, so please bear with me. It's about an elderly blind woman and her non-irascible, non-vexatious and not even remotely cranky way of dealing with adversity. Here is the (anonymous) story, in case you missed it.

She is 92 years old, petite, well poised, and proud. She is fully dressed each morning by eight o'clock, with her hair fashionably coifed, and her makeup perfectly applied, in spite of the fact she is legally blind. Today she has moved to a nursing home. Her husband of 70 years recently passed away, making this move necessary. After many hours of waiting patiently in the lobby of the nursing home, where I am employed, she smiled sweetly when told her room was ready.

As she maneuvered her walker to the elevator, I provided a visual description of her tiny room, including the eyelet curtains that had been hung on her window. 'I love it,' she stated with the enthusiasm of an eight-year-old having just been presented with a new puppy. 'Mrs. Jones, you haven't seen the room ... just wait,' I said.

Then she spoke these words that I will never forget: 'That does not have anything to do with it,' she gently replied. 'Happiness is something you decide on ahead of time. Whether I like my room or not, does not depend on how the furniture is arranged. It is how I arrange my mind. I have already decided to love it. It is a decision I make every morning when I wake up. I have a choice. I can spend the day in bed recounting the difficulty I have with the parts of my body that no longer work, or I can get out of bed and be thankful for the ones that do work. Each day is a gift, and as long as my eyes open, I will focus on the new day and all of the happy memories I have stored away...just for this time in my life."

Aw shucks, isn't that sweet? Doesn't it just make you want to be a little more agreeable, positive and predisposed to looking on the bright side? What does it matter if the story is untrue, as it surely is?

Well, of course it matters. But, in this case, it shows that attitude is key, and the focus is to develop skills over time that turn difficult people into agreeable folks who are just a little bit more like the heroine in this little morality tale about the extremes of looking on the bright side of life. Furthermore, it's a good contrast between lovable and obnoxious people!

Who among us has not, at one time or another, probably today, had to deal with a "difficult" person? The experience must be universal. Would that everyone could be more like the sweet 92 year-old in the story. Alas, we know reality is otherwise. Knowing that, it might be wise to search for and test out a few uniquely wellness ways to deal effectively with such individuals.

I started such explorations years ago because I was receiving so much mail asking for advice about how to deal with obnoxious neighbors, co-workers and friends of friends. Here is an example of one such message:

"Dr. Ardell, one of our co-workers is driving us nuts. We work in a large company with many departments. People in each department have more than enough work to do (our company believes in staffing lightly) and the jobs are very specialized. Not only do most people have advanced educations, but each role takes quite a lot of training. This person frequently makes last minute (or late) demands, continually operates in crisis mode and not only issues unreasonable requests but frequently accompanies these with instructions on how we might proceed to perform the work for which she is being paid! She is usually wrong in analyzing procedures and laying out instructions; in addition, her demands are delivered with the allusion that she is much more intelligent than the dullards she is forced to deal with and if we weren't all so stupid and would just follow her lead, we could be a lot more efficient. Other factors in the equation include her lack of attention to her own job details and her reluctance to cooperate with other people. What do you suggest as proactive, wellness-oriented behavior when dealing with her?"

This sounded to me like a situation for Superwellnessman.

Where to start? I pondered it and I pondered it. Then I pondered some more.

What would I recommend? Then, I had a revelation—introduce the difficult person to the 92 year-old blind lady! Unfortunately, that was not possible, since the latter was surely fictional, like me being a Superwellnessman of advice.

But, eventually, some ideas here and there came to mind.

How about a national database of really nice people by neighborhood listed throughout America? When an obnoxious person, or just irascible, vexatious and cranky seniors become a public nuisance, dial a number for a certified nice person who would visit the public nuisance character and, in no time at all, some of the latter's niceness would rub off.

Seriously, difficult seniors and irascible, vexatious and cranky folks of all ages are commonplace. They need more love, understanding and interactions with clever folks who bring out the best in them and turn them around, little by little, over time. Not everyone can be reformed, of course, but many can be improved and toned down, and you might be just the person to serve as change agent for spreading niceness—by doing a bit of the artful toning and improving.

I myself have to deal with a difficult employee, and I work alone. It's tough all over. Sometimes the greatest of challenges is to deal not with the other person who of course is the sole cause of all the difficulty, but to temper your own reactions to a difficult (or impossible!) person. This is always a lot easier than efforts, however skilled, to change someone. After all, if such an individual were "reform-able," someone probably would have succeeded in doing so by now.

In the case described by the letter writer, above, I suggested that, if all else fails, desperation measures could be employed, including a few that are legal and entail no violence. I sympathized with the victim's plight, and asked if she tried humor? Maybe turning the tables, practical jokes—that sort of thing? Turns out nobody had thought of doing anything like that, and after I suggested, nobody thought much of it then, either. But, I had other tips left to put forward. After all, not everyone has a well-developed sense of mirth, an ability to appreciate the ludicrous and absurdly incongruous. Some become flummoxed by juxtaposition and surprise, which by the way are other key elements in humor dynamics.

Next I tried a little humor of my own, asking about the possibility that the woman causing all the trouble might be right, that is, everything WOULD be a lot more efficient if everyone would just follow her lead! This was seen as most amusing. But, I still needed to come up with something useful. So, I offered these tips. I hope a few will help you manage difficult seniors.

- Try a charm offensive. Whenever the obnoxious person is, well, obnoxious, try a little theater, preferably in a conspiracy with others. Whoop it up. Suggest that she is absolutely right and more diligent efforts will be made to meet her high but enlightened standards. This probably won't work, but it might be fun for a while and get your mind off the stress the person causes.

- Call a meeting, with an outside facilitator. Brainstorm ways to deal with the issues and to have a better environment for getting the job done and done well, while supporting each other as much as possible. Be sure to invite the difficult person to the meeting!

- Lobby the bosses to promote this woman to a high position in the company, out of your work area. Open an office in Australia. See that she becomes the director of this keen new division.

- After all these reasonable efforts to modify the problem-person fail, then it might be time for a down-to-earth, matter-of-fact confrontation. If a united group of co-workers lays it out, specifying what she's doing and how it's affecting them, a desirable outcome has to be she'll quit.

- There are probably other possibilities (exorcism?) but I can't think of any more at the moment. If none of this helps, take comfort in the knowledge that everyone has a right to be a twit now and then, though some surely do abuse the privilege.

I shared this tip with Rick Clark, one of my philosopher buddies, an irascible senior himself who sniffed and replied, "My advice would be slightly different: I say avoid all irascible, vexatious, cranky people— particularly seniors. Forgive me, but I think this is better advice. I mean, I know that if I were someone else I'd certainly avoid me. Plus there's another good reason to follow this alternate plan: There's always the chance that God might eventually come to His almighty senses and start tossing lighting bolts after all, and you don't want to be in the vicinity of those cranky folks when that happens."

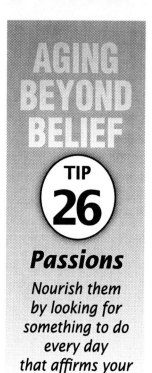

AGING BEYOND BELIEF

TIP
26

Passions

Nourish them by looking for something to do every day that affirms your "zest for life"

*T*hink about ways to get paid, if only a little, for doing what you enjoy. Take your time about it—the search for activities that deliver such feelings of zest or exuberance may take decades. Such feelings are often associated with true passions, avocations that can define who you really are or seek to become. The payoff for such pursuits in not fame or fortune, but the doing, the satisfactions from the pursuit of your vision. No matter your age, there is time to do this. The payoffs are often immediate.

Whatever the final outcome, the experience of fashioning your art, over time while developing passion for some outcomes will be of consequence, to you. If you love what you're doing, it isn't work any more. It's purpose and play, all rolled into one. Yes, you be the sole judge of what qualifies as "zestful" enough to count. How hard can it be to spend a portion of every day searching for a more joyful, creative outlook? Don't worry about talent if you have any interest at all in painting, singing, dancing or whatever. Do what appeals to you. For many, such a thing is often of an artistic nature. Most of the time, others will make a big fuss about it, especially if you're old enough. But, that's a bonus, even if you enjoy public acclaim (not everyone does). More important, you'll have a good time doing something creative and, of course, zestful.

For years I was "hot on the trail" of added zest in my own life. No, I was not seeking to know how the brain stores memories (how knowledge is represented in the human mind), nor was I trying to work out a solid state theory explaining superconductivity that allows electricity to flow unimpeded at relatively warm temperatures—a form of electronic perpetual motion. What, then? You're probably thinking, "I know, Don was looking for the missing matter in the universe" (physicists have calculated that the total mass in the cosmos is 10 times what we've been able to observe) or an answer to the puzzle whether life might have evolved elsewhere in the universe?" No, I have not spent any time seeking zest by exploring these matters. What, then?

Do you give up?

It has to do with taking a new look at a negative phenomenon, namely, the powerful but poorly regarded process known as denial! (You seldom hear a good word for denial, a term meaning self-delusion, for the very good reason that it is usually manifested in persons a bit out of contact with reality. Where's the zest in denial? Well, around this time, a good friend and very serious athlete of 60+ years advised that his oxygen uptake had been tested, but he was sorely disappointed with the result. He concluded that the relatively low score indicated that age was overtaking his best efforts to stay young. I shot back a demurrer, insisting that the results were misinterpreted, that the test taker was biased, that the instruments malfunctioned and/or that the very concept of such a test was flawed! He immediately felt better, recognizing the scientific validity of my instincts. I told my colleague in Australia, Grant Donovan, about this and he replied, as follows: "Thanks for the interesting medical report about our mutual friend, and your explanation of the situation. I'm happy to see you're now doing denials for other people. It might be time to set it up as a business. Some people do readings, Shirley does connections and Don does denials. I bet there's big money to be made denying other people are old, overweight, having affairs, committing mayhem and so on. I think you should create a Denials Center at SeekWellness.com."

Well, by that time I knew I was really getting close to the breakthrough and thus feeling pretty zestful. But, I needed a word for the kind of denial I would promote—and a little bit of plausible evidence (even if only slightly plausible evidence.)

No sooner did I start thinking along these lines than along comes an expert who thinks self-delusion contributes to marital accord! That's right—psychologist Benjamin Karney of the University of Florida says people who can use their memories selectively tend to believe that their marriage is better now than in the past. The key is to recall and give credence to the good stuff and consciously learn to forget the not so good. In short, it's healthy to delude ourselves a bit for AUI purposes. So much for Sir Walter Scott's (1771-1832) line about a tangled web! ("Oh, what a tangled web we weave, when first we practice to deceive." This is also attributed to Shakespeare, but Scott seems the critic's choice of first author of the line.) According to an article in the Miami Herald about the study Karney conducted over a 20-year period, it's good to be able to tell yourself a story you like to believe. Karney wrote that it's okay not to be accurate about the past if it makes you feel better about the present. Just so, I say. Selective positive memories often make the difference between happiness and misery. This applies to childhood memories, the way you think about your job and profession, how you view your performances as a lover—the works.

Politicians often seek "plausible deniability" when seeking to pull a fast one on their constituents and the rest of the country. My zest-inducing breakthrough tip should henceforth be known as "positive affirmal." It's AFFIRMING, not DENYING. It's much better than simple denial or plausible deniability—provided of course you know that you are only fooling yourself temporarily for the purpose of adding zest. Do this in the context of organizing your affairs so as to better AUI—of wellness lifestyles.

*D*oing so just might help you experience more of it, more often, which is a very nice thing. Study the literature, the art and the science of happiness. Learn more about what great thinkers and ordinary thinkers have written about it, how it is studied and ideas for boosting your levels of it. The more you know about what happiness is and how it works, the more likely you are to experience its pleasures. Humor, fun and joy are among some the most obvious forms of happiness. Laughter and assorted pleasures strengthen the immune system, metabolize bad vibes and serve to make your everyday life a little richer.

Happiness is shaped by three factors: genetics, circumstances and choices. The first two categories, according to findings from the emerging field of "Positive Psychology," are estimated to account for 50 and 12 percent of happiness, respectively. The rest is up for grabs!

More to Happiness Than Meets the Eye

Become something of an expert on the science of happiness

The factors listed under genetics (DNA) and circumstances (for example, age, sex, economic status, education, etc.) create a "setpoint" for almost two-thirds of your happiness. This leaves a substantial percentage as "wiggle room for happiness." That your cue—make the most of it.

Edward Newton (The Book Collecting Game, 1928) said, "happiness is to be very busy with the unimportant." Ogden Nash, in his inimitable style, wrote, "There is only one way to achieve happiness on this terrestrial ball, And that is to have either a clear conscience, or none at all."

Seligman and Royzman ("Happiness: The Three Traditional Theories") use the word "hedonism" to describe theories on the nature of happiness. Hedonism is described as a feeling outlook. A happy life is one of maximum pleasure, minimum pain. Its intellectual inspiration is utilitarianism, rooted in the works of Jeremy Betham. Desire is a matter of getting what you want. I suppose everyone would be happy holding this construct provided he/she did not want very much. Desire theory places the realization of whatever the desire is (to rule the world, be elected mayor or whatever) above that of experiencing pleasure, though one might assume that achieving a heart's desire would be rather pleasurable. Otherwise, what would motivate the desire? Wittgenstein is cited as a writer who, by extolling truth, illumination, struggle and purity, contributed to our understanding of happiness. Happiness is influenced by "career accomplishments, friendship, relief from pain, material comforts, civic spirit, beauty, education, love, knowledge and good conscience."

Seligman identifies three distinct traditions or elements of "authentic happiness," namely, the pleasures of a pleasant life, the engagement of the good life and the meaningful life. All are subjective, though Seligman would have us believe the latter can be partly objective. The meaningful life is simply a term for the wellness dimension of meaning and purpose, in my view. Seligman's description of it mirrors that of Frankl. The bottom line is this: Happiness ensues from "belonging to and serving what is larger and more worthwhile," it does not follow from seeking "the self's pleasures and desires." Reach out and be of service—this is the surest way to happiness.

In *Stumbling on Happiness* (Alfred A. Knopf, 2006), Harvard psychologist Daniel Gilbert connects scientific research in varied fields (psychology, cognitive neuroscience, philosophy and economics) to explain happiness or its absence, explaining among other things why we "misconceive our tomorrows and misestimate our satisfactions."

Of course, all these terms interrelate and complement each other. The pleasant life is somewhat hedonistic, the good life is filled with desire and the meaningful life must encompass happiness. Naturally, the forms happiness takes vary considerably within individuals and cultures.

Exercising Critical Faculties

Develop and use reason by practicing good thinking skills

*S*tart by being a bit skeptical about some of the things you believe. It's bloody time to root out your own dysfunctional notions, faulty assumptions, prejudices, biases and essentially loony misconceptions. Assuming that, like me, you might be harboring a few, here and there. Flaws in reasoning interfere with your ability to function well in the later years, just as earlier in life. We tend to distrust information at odds with beliefs we prefer to maintain! Consider shaping a learning environment that prizes skepticism, doubt, evidence, critical thinking and reason. In particular, verify claims through independent third party sources. Give little credence to ads and testimonials from persons with vested interests. A good book for learning more about this tip is *Don't Believe Everything You Think* by Thomas Kida (Prometheus Books, 2006).

One of the biggest dangers to effective decision-making is peer pressure. Resolve not to cave every time "go along to get along" pressure is applied. Otherwise, you will be seen an easy mark. That is the first rule of critical thinking—hold your ground until YOU are convinced about the best course.

1. Don't cave—be alert to and quick to sidestep peer pressures.

2. Don't believe everything you think, in fact, be suspicious of most of what you think. After all, you have probably been exposed to a mountain of nonsense over the years, and a lot of it probably got past your poorly developed, suppressed doo doo detectors.

3. Don't hold on to weird ideas. If you embrace beliefs at odds with science, and who doesn't save a few unusual characters

among us, subject these superstitions to critical scrutiny. The goal is to lighten the nonsense load that will weigh you down. Examples of absolute nonsense that many otherwise semi-sensible people embrace include such foolishness as homeopathy, ESP, astrology, psychokinesis, haunted houses, reincarnation, devil possession, clairvoyance, telepathy, communication with the dead and therapeutic touch. There's much more but this will get you started. Eradicating weird notions is a big job for most people—get started now.

4. Don't fall for anecdotes. Develop a healthy respect for statistics and rely more on data than stories. Data enable decision processes that are more objective, unemotional and conducive to sound decision-making. Anecdotes are usually ladled with bias, partial information, rumor and/or urban lore, plus self-interest. Be especially cynical about stories that support what you already believe, another common thought process tendency that is quite dysfunctional. Pay as much attention to information that contradicts what you want to believe as to information that supports your expectations. Consider: Things don't cause feelings; we attach feelings to events.

5. Don't think everything that happens has profound or other meaning. If you think "there's a reason for everything," get your head examined. Just kidding —that's harsh. Just having a little fun here. No, seriously, this "reason for everything" cliché is a grotesquery, a truly twisted notion. Chance and coincidence play a major role in everyone's life. Because evolution made us causal-seeking animals and religions led us to believe the gods intervene in the minutiae of our affairs, we are programmed to look for meaning in everything. These cultural norms are worth resisting. Do NOT accept associations, connections and links when none exist.

6. Don't oversimplify or rely on your memory to excess. Yes, life is complex and we have to streamline decisions to

save time and effort. This can't be helped but be alert to a tendency to overlook important information in the rush to judgment. Memories are unreliable—they change over time in response to current beliefs, expectations, suggestive questioning and dying brain cells.

7. Avoid overconfidence in your thinking processes. As Bertrand Russell advised, "the fundamental cause of trouble in the world today is that the stupid are cocksure while the intelligent are full of doubt."

A critical mindset is needed for AUI of a wellness lifestyle. Another revealing book is *Why People Believe Weird Things* by Michael Shermer. He describes a deficiency called "confirmational bias" causes people to become "skilled at defending beliefs they arrived at for non-smart reasons." This seems profoundly true, and explains why many seniors and others sometimes think poorly and behave foolishly. Yet another favorite source I recommend is *The Skeptics Guide to the Universe*, a weekly Podcast talkshow produced by the New England Skeptical Society and the James Randi Educational Foundation (JREF). Here you will find topics from the world of the paranormal, fringe science and controversial claims, all dissected from a scientific point of view.

The following data on irrationality in America was reported in the National Science Foundation's biennial report in 2002 and according to a 2005 update, the extent of irrational beliefs increased in recent years (See Newport F., Strausberg M. 201. "Americans' belief in psychic and paranormal phenomena is up over last decade," *Gallup Poll News Service*, 8 June. www.gallup.com):

- 30 percent of adult Americans believe space vehicles from other civilizations (UFOs) are practicing takeoffs and landings in the US;

- 60 percent believe in extra-sensory perception (ESP);

- 40 percent believe in astrology;

- 32 percent believe in lucky numbers;

- 70 percent accept magnetic therapy as scientific; and

- 88 percent accept alternative medicine.

- The one statistic that, in my opinion, explains all the other data is this one: 70 percent of Americans still do not understand the scientific process. While none of us goes through every step in this process before making decisions day in and day out, an understanding of basic concepts of probability, the experimental method and hypothesis testing does inform our views about UFO sightings, ESP, astrology, numerology, magnetic therapy, claims for alternative medicine and other odd beliefs. All of which reminds me once again of the merits of promoting the elements of logic (the "BS detector") that Carl Sagan described in his masterwork, *The Demon-Haunted World.*

A wellness remedy for confirmational bias entails the practice and mastery of these and other thinking skills. Why do so many people become accustomed to "defending beliefs they arrived at for non-smart reasons," as Shermer suggests? A partial list of factors includes cultural reinforcements over time along with "genetic predisposition, parental predilection, sibling influence, peer pressure, educational experience and life impressions." All these factors contribute to our beliefs and, once we have them, we "sort through the body of data and select those that most confirm what we already believe, and ignore or rationalize away those that do not." That is what is called "confirmation bias" and it might explain why so many believe, contrary to science and reason, in UFO sightings, ESP, astrology, numerology, magnetic therapy and the claims for alternative medicine.

Part of the wellness remedy is to devote more attention to how science works, along with the practice of critical thinking. This seems even more significant than teaching students current theories favored by science. HOW science works might be more consequential for people struggling with poor logic than WHAT science has discovered. Seniors can apply what they know about science to reject pseudo-scientific ideas and a smorgasbord of false claims. To overcome confirmation bias, it seems more important to learn HOW rather than just WHAT to think.

Good luck thinking.

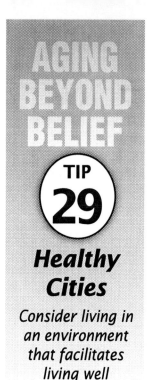

AGING BEYOND BELIEF

TIP

29

Healthy Cities

Consider living in an environment that facilitates living well

*E*ach year, the US Centers for Disease Control and Prevention (CDC) publishes America's Health: State Health Rankings. The Rankings report contains recommendations for community leaders for shaping environments most conducive to optimal health. If you are a senior with the mobility to live where you can, this publication contains invaluable data for making travel plans, if necessary.

Want to guess which state came out #1, that is, healthiest of all states in the US? How about #50? I won't keep you in suspense—Minnesota ranked as America's healthiest state. Let's hear it for the gopher state, which has as it's official bird the Common Loon (gavia immer), a creature with a 600 million year history making it one of this good earth's oldest living bird species. According to the official website of this most healthy of all American states, there are about 12,000 loons (as opposed to loonies, an entirely different species) in Minnesota. Loons are large black-and-white birds with long black bills. Clumsy on land, they are excellent divers, underwater swimmers, and high-speed flyers.

Of course, I digress; let's get back to the rankings.

Minnesota's position at the top will come as no surprise to followers of the Rankings report, since it has been either number one or two since 1990. New Hampshire, which has occasionally traded places with Minnesota as number one in the rankings since 1990, is second this year. Vermont is third, followed by Hawaii, Utah and Massachusetts.

At the other end of the ranks is Louisiana, the nation's least healthy state before the arrival of Katrina and not likely to have moved up since. Mississippi, Tennessee, South Carolina and Arkansas round out the five least healthy states. My own home state of Florida is 42nd, nothing to brag about.

Minnesota's strengths include low death rates for cardiovascular disease and premature deaths, as well as a low rate of citizens without health insurance. It also scored high for its support of public health and low rates of children in poverty, infant mortality, occupational fatalities and high rates of high school graduation. On the other hand, even the healthiest state has problems, namely, a high prevalence of obesity (23.0 percent) and low access to adequate prenatal care (only 76.0 percent of pregnant women in Minnesota received adequate prenatal care). Of course, most of these factors are of little consequence to those of us AUI of wellness lifestyles. Still, it's good if others around us are enjoying good health.

Louisiana is 50th this year, a position it has held for all but one of the fifteen years of the CDC reports. It is among the bottom five states on six of 18 key health measures, namely premature death rate, infant mortality rate, rate of cancer deaths, percentage of children in poverty, rate of uninsured population and prevalence of smoking. It also ranks in the bottom ten states for five other measures. Again, all before Katrina. Pitiful.

The Ranking report concludes with five categories of action recommendations—all of which makes great sense for seniors:

- Learn about your own health—blood pressure, cholesterol, body mass index, etc.— and identify your own risk factors— smoking, exercise, genetic, occupational, etc. Learn about nutrition and food labeling, understand the role and value of regular exercise and preventive care and practice good personal hygiene.

- Access the resources available to you: public parks and trails for exercise; stores for fresh fruits and vegetables; your healthcare provider for preventive care; public health services for information, tools and statistics; schools for education and training; and community and church groups for social engagement and personal fulfillment.

- Participate in public health education and screening programs, join support programs to help you with your problems, and implement your regular fitness and wellness program.

- Change your own behaviors, take charge and understand yourself, identify inhibitors to personal change, identify resources that can help you change, set a plan and then do it. Specific behaviors to nurture include regular physical activity, healthier weight, good nutrition, no tobacco use or substance abuse, responsible sexual behavior, mental health well-being, safe and injury-free activities, regular immunizations and routine preventative health care.

- Teach and mentor others, especially your own and the community's children. Set an example of sound health behaviors; discuss healthy living and your personal plans and habits. Be active. Share through your example.

While the Rankings report is a fine resource, I question if the data used by the CDC really identify the healthiest states. The data compiled for the annual report are appropriate for identifying and ranking the unhealthiest states, but measures of dysfunction (for example, death rates from various diseases, premature deaths, health insurance levels, children in poverty, infant mortality, occupational fatalities and high school graduation rates) do not reflect the presence of advanced states of well-being as would a selection of indices for positive functioning.

Perhaps the CDC will evolve and in time promote wellness awareness, as well as disease and dysfunction assessment. If that happens, we might look forward to reports of well-being, both physical and mental, regarding genuine achievements on a state-by-state basis. This requires the CDC to identify fitness and nutrition measures, as well as others of positive health and life quality.

"What measures might these be?" The significant resources of the CDC will be needed to make that determination, after some period of study and public input; but I would imagine the selected indicators would reflect the extent that populations are happy, the degree adverse consequences of aging are inhibited with proactive lifestyle habits, as well as indicators reflecting satisfying relationships, ample enjoyment of humor and play levels, the capacity of people for critical thinking and the extent to which residents experience meaning and purpose in their lives. That would be a good starter set, and the kind of data that would enable a more accurate picture of genuine health than the current collection of morbidity, mortality and perturbation levels.

Without such positive information, we won't really know if Minnesota, New Hampshire, Vermont, Hawaii, Utah and Massachusetts are in fact any "weller" in the positive sense of health than the seemingly backwater states of the south. In fact, there is nothing to keep civic boosters in Louisiana and other bottom-of-the-health-barrel states from deluding themselves with spurious claims for being truly healthier than they really are, based on seriously bogus criteria (for example, "We're # 1 in college football and tattooed fans of NASCAR")!

However, please do not let all this detail distract you from what should be the two main messages of this tip, neither of which I have made, until now. The first is to congratulate the CDC for its role in producing the Rankings report for fifteen years—it is an excellent work as far as it goes, and will pave the way for wellness rankings at some point in the future. The second is that no matter what ranking your state obtained, you can be number one in terms of living the healthiest, most satisfying possible quality of life within your power. You can live a wellness lifestyle in Louisiana as well as Minnesota, or anywhere else. It may be a little more challenging in some states than others, but it will always be your choice, wherever you are. It's just easier in some locations than others, so if you are able to live wherever you like in your senior years, pick a healthy place, other things being the same.

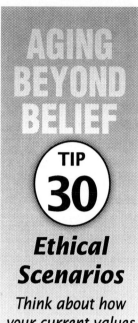

Ethical Scenarios

Think about how your current values might come into play under extreme situations

At the beginning of 2007, the whole world, it seemed, was talking about Wesley Autrey, a 50 year-old construction worker from Harlem who saved a man who had fallen onto subway tracks in New York City. Mr. Autrey covered the victim's body with his own as the train passed over. Both lived—and Autrey deservedly became one of the most feted humans on the planet, not just for 15 minutes but for at least as many days. His appearance on CBS' "Late Show with David Letterman" the next day was a sensation on YouTube. Thinking of this recent episode led me to reflect on my response years ago to the Titanic exhibition at a local museum.

I was fascinated by the memorabilia recovered from the sea floor, including china, glass bottles, photos, jewelry, washbasins, a pen, a lamp, slippers and eyeglasses. A bracelet, the name "Amy" spelled out in gemstones and never claimed, seemed to stand out. I wondered, "Was Amy one of the 1,523 of the 2,228 passengers and crew who perished, or did she make it and, if so, what became of her?" The most gripping moment for me was standing on the recreated wooden deck, with portals, benches and rails. It's late evening on the night of the sinking and the sky is painted just as it was that evening, filled with the exact same stars the passengers would have seen. You can see the looming iceberg, shown in high relief. I felt a lump in my throat, much like the feeling earlier in downtown Dallas, standing in a museum above Dealey Plaza where an assassin perched on November 22, 1963 in the sixth floor window of the former Texas School Book Depository.

Soon after my visit to the Titanic exhibit, I came upon an article based on a survey conducted by a Pennsylvania newspaper on the occasion of the 80th anniversary of the ship's sinking. The survey showed that contemporary males would in no way behave as gallantly, as chivalrously as did the "real" men of 1912. Naturally, this survey provided a rich treasure of material for columnists and talk show hosts—and added new spice to the always-contentious modern issue of how to treat older people, as well as male-female rights and privileges. In most of the discussions, nearly everyone, including older folks, seems to agree that in such a situation, the old should step aside for the young, if space on the lifeboats is limited. This has not made me any likelier to go on North Atlantic or other cruises and, the older I get, the LESS likely such cruises tend to appeal to me. (Unless I were guaranteed access to my own seaworthy watercraft brought along for me alone, just in case.)

Ask yourself a few ethical questions, if only for ethical inventory purposes.

Should seniors stay behind to save others? At what age, exactly, does an older person lose a place on a scarce lifeboat? What if you are fit and youthful looking at 69 and can easily pass for 60, but somebody in charge put the eligibility age at 65. Do you fess up, or move gracefully toward the lifeboat, with a youthful bounce in your stride?

Never mind if men should defer to women, or what to do with the physically challenged (and HOW physically challenged one should be to be favored or sacrificed), the punk rocker or the fool with the ghetto blaster? Where might lines be drawn? What kinds of calls would you want to make or, in the present case, simply defend in a situational ethics-type parlor game?

Play this game for a short time and you realize that there is no rule or norm in place for contemporary Titanic situations and, interestingly, there is little consensus that there should be!

Of course, you also realize how important it is that there be enough lifeboats. But, in varied life situations, there are never enough lifeboats, when the latter term is but a metaphor for goods and services that are scarce and subject to supply and demand.

Maybe the chances are not so great that you will ever be on the North Atlantic in a sinking cruise ship with too few lifeboats listening to the band play *Nearer My God To Thee*, looking around and wondering, OK, let's see now, who gets to go first around here? Nevertheless, you can better understand your own values and ponder the need for a little tweaking by doing a little imagining of this kind every so often. If nothing else, it will give you something to be grateful for, namely, that you were not on board a very big, sinking ship in 1912.

Everyone interested in optimal function must be curious about her own values. Who would not wonder, standing on the deck of the model Titanic at this exhibit, how he or she would respond in a tight situation. What emphasis would you place upon chivalry, loyalty, morality and the like for insight into how you would deal with or react in a life-threatening situation?

Just whom do you look out for, not just in hypothetical life or death sacrifices but in your day- to-day actions that affect the quality of life of those around you?

The answers here are actually not all that different from those that faced John Jacob Astor (he declined a rowboat seat), Bruce Ismay (he took one), Amy (who lost her bracelet, and probably her life) and the others on that fateful night 94 years ago.

Whatever your opinion of traditional chivalry, modern feminism or women's rights in an egalitarian society, and whatever your sex or sexual preference, chances are that the only kind of ethics that will guide your actions in a New Titanic situation are "situational" in nature. Just like the one Wesley Autrey had to deal with in our time.

In our extraordinarily diverse society, don't expect a lot of consensus on such ethical choices, but try to make peace with the man or woman you have to face each morning in the mirror. Situational ethics may not be a favored topic for contemporary preachers but, if you don't know what you believe and what's worth dying for, if anything, what else can you rely upon in times that invite great courage, if not sacrifice?

"Know thyself" is easier repeated than achieved. A few minutes on the deck of the Titanic, even a model of the original, is a sobering experience. It makes one think, about a lot of things, not least of all the meaning of life, the nature of heroism, bravery, love and even one's own commitment to rationality, convention and situational ethics.

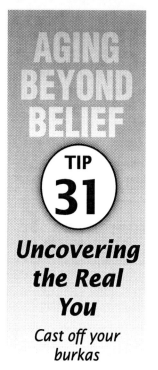

AGING
BEYOND
BELIEF

TIP

31

Uncovering the Real You

Cast off your burkas

I recently spoke at a company retreat in Lake Tahoe, CA. After my introduction (flowery and much enhanced—it's not so important to write your own speech, but it's crucial to do your own introduction), I swept into the room with a bit of pomp if not circumstance, or vice-versa. I made my way to the stage wearing a full burka, as Pat Benatar's voice singing "Hit Me With Your Best Shot! Why Don't You Hit Me With Your Best Shot! Hit Me With Your Best Shot! Fire Away!" entertained all present. You get everyone's undivided attention when you set the stage for a speech in this fashion.

Here is what I said, initially, more or less, after standing wordlessly at the lectern for a moment after the music stopped. The pregnant pause complete, I began my talk:

Good morning. I'm here to describe the role of fitness and wellness in shaping the quality of your life and the success of your business. I will discuss exercise, nutrition, happiness and finding meaning and purpose from work and in the rest of your life.

You might be thinking, 'Is this guy going to stand up there, his face and body totally covered in a burka, and expect us to listen to him for an hour and a half? He must be kidding.' "

Being so intuitive, I did indeed sense what everyone was thinking (see above). I said, "I can guess what you're thinking. 'Is this guy going to stand up there, his face and body totally covered in a burka, and expect us to listen to him for an hour and a half? He must be kidding.'"

If I did that, that is, if I remained here wearing this burka for the entire time, you would be unable to appreciate:

- My expressive eyes.

- My winning smile.

- My impressive hairstyle.

- My mesmerizing eye contact.

I would not want you to miss out on any of that. Therefore, I shall cast off my burka! (At this point, the burka was removed with a flourish, to much applause and merriment.)

Now I want to ask you to cast off YOUR burkas!

I know, nobody is wearing a burka. I realize you do not dress in a burka to go to work, when you drive, when you party or when you exercise. I'm quite sure that you NEVER wear a burka, in fact, I doubt if anyone does or ever would own such a thing, let alone wear it.

I'm talking about burkas metaphorically. You probably believe, as I do, that the burka represents an imposition of dogma over common sense and reflects the oppression of women. At least, that's my KINDEST explanation. Naturally, YOU would not wear a burka, nor would anyone in your family do so, unless of course you were raised in a culture where such a monstrosity of attire is the norm. You are a liberated person, free to dress, speak, write, go and do as you please. However, you almost surely would benefit from casting off your metaphorical burkas. These metaphorical burkas take the form of dysfunctional customs, traditions, norms and unexamined rituals. Things that you might have long taken for granted might be covering your true, best possible self, cloaking your potentials and obscuring your vision. That's why I suggest you cast off your burkas, specifically the subtle kind that obscure your view of best possibilities.

Well, there you have it. The opening of my keynote. I think this opening was well received, and I would like to think the rest was good for them, as well. The talk certainly was fun to deliver.

In any event, I offer the burka metaphor as a tip for you. It should be of interest, especially if YOU have any metaphorical burkas over your head, covering your eyes from a clear view of the big picture.

Think of a senior you know or have read about who adapted quite well to one or more demands of added years. Think of how this person would bring dignity, panache and/or flair to the challenge you face. This simple mental process might elicit some good ideas for you, in your situation.

What Would Your Exemplar Do?

Consider a hero or two

Epictetus (c.55–c.135 C.E.) had a few interesting ideas that might apply to a consideration of this tip. He urged his students to live the philosophic life, which he called "eudaimonia" (meaning 'happiness' or 'flourishing') via the pursuit of reason. For Stoics, this meant living virtuously in accordance with nature. However, he also advised against the hazards of a dull nature. "What might that be?" you ask? Too little attention to love, sex and belonging, esteem and the need to find fulfillment in life—at all ages.

In a crisis, of course, survival comes first. Even here, an AUI orientation will serve admirably, as a strong constitution boosts prospects for survival and full recovery. If depravations are to be endured, better to start out in a state of excellent health than weakened by dissolution. In top form, one will last longer than if overweight, underfit, out of shape, immunity compromised or lacking in rational survival skills. Such skills include personal responsibility, stress management, resiliency, emotional intelligence, critical thinking and an absolute devotion to common decencies. Common decencies are always evident, particularly when the shooting starts, the waters rise, supplies run out. That is when compassion, kindness, courage and a willingness to be of service appear as true hallmarks of heroic value systems.

No need to look back thousands of years for heroes, however. In good times and during crises, there are those around us who do things they need not do, in service to others. Think of those who inspire you who, under pressure, would do the right and noble thing. (Recall tip # 30 concerning situational ethics.)

A wellness mindset is a positive, enjoyable approach to living well, with panache and style. You are not disposed to follow experts who urge restrictions or limits on your options.

A few years ago, the *Wall Street Journal* published a piece entitled, "Top 10 Health Mistakes." It listed medical errors older people commonly make, based upon interviews done with about 500 seniors.

I reinterpreted this advice, making the information more upbeat and consistent with a wellness orientation. I think the information is best presented in a positive manner, with a touch of humor and irreverence. Such a spin is, in my view, more likely to motivate seniors (and others) to take proactive initiatives. I'll demonstrate this assertion with a rework of the ten health mistakes described, converting them into ten positive messages.

A Positive Spin on Grim Warnings

Reinterpret droll, negative health messages

In the examples given, sentence "A" states the mistakes, as described by the medical experts. Sentence "B," by contrast, is a wellness way of expressing the same idea, not as a mistake commonly made but as a guideline to consider.

Make no mistake—these "mistakes" are serious issues, omissions and lost opportunities. However, my sense is that the same messages can be delivered in upbeat, positive ways. Better to stress the advantages of taking initiatives than to inadvertently browbeat old people for overlooking common sense precautions.

Check out the contrasts. "A" is the common expert approach that seems like a scolding; "B" is a more artful way to make the same point, as a gentle but persuasive suggestion.

1. Driving

   A. The mistake is to drive after senility sets in.

   B. Let others do the driving—sit back and enjoy the ride! Driving is a drag. It's stressful, dangerous and expensive. Besides, now that you are so old, if you get in a crash, everyone will assume it's because you are senile! Avoid the aggravation—let others do the work. You have earned the right to be chauffeured about.

2. Slowing down

   A. The mistake is to deny that you have deteriorated (e.g., failure to utilize hearing aids, wear dentures).

   B. Geological change over time shapes mountain peaks—and time changes you, too! You live in a modern age—take advantage of technological aides that can keep you functionally younger, longer.

3. Disclosure

   A. The mistake is not giving relevant information to caregivers (The example given was not telling your doctor you can't perform sexually as well as you'd like. Well, what guy CAN perform as well as he'd LIKE? At ANY age!)

   B. Doctors are paid to hear about your intimate problems of a personal nature. Give them an earful! Make your symptoms sound much worse than they are, just for fun. Then tell the real story—your problems won't seem so bad. The fact is you should get your money's worth by having the doctor evaluate all concerns, real and imagined, to see if there might be larger problems, or maybe no problems at all, thus freeing you to live it up and take more chances in enjoyable ways.

4. Treatment protocols

   A. The mistake is not asking enough questions to fully understand what should be done.

B. Get the doctor to write down his/her recommendations in plain English—or whatever language you prefer. Don't let the doctor get away with using big words that confuse you.

5. Home design

A. The mistake is not being cautious, especially about preventing falls.

B. Become an "ecospace design engineer!" Bring in family members, friends and others to give advice on ways to make your home more conducive to wellness, so you can exercise more and eat better—and avoid falls and other hazards. Exercising more and eating wisely will strengthen your bones and muscles; redesigning living spaces will protect against accidents that could interfere with your active lifestyle.

6. Medications

A. The mistake is not getting detailed instruction and insuring that medical personnel know what drugs you are already taking.

B. The best drugs are those that are absolutely necessary and that do not create other problems besides those they are designed to remedy. Make sure your doctor knows what you are taking and that YOU know why and how to use the medication. In this way, you can protect your energy level and stay alert, the better to enjoy yourself.

7. A primary doctor

A. The mistake is not having one to oversee everything.

B. If you keep your medical records up-to-date, you can "seize the day" each time you encounter a doctor or other provider by insuring that he/she knows your history and, more important, your high expectations for an active, wellness lifestyle. In that spirit, the provider will appreciate that you are serious about staying well and avoid the common mistake of over— medicalizing you just because you are an older person.

8. Paying attention

   A. The mistake is ignoring warning signs of one problem or another.

   B. Ask about warning signs, but also ask about options for making positive advances in your health status. Be sure the doctor is aware of how well you are so the focus is not entirely on looking for bad news. The good news about your strengths and assets (good health habits) should be taken into account at all checkups.

9. Prevention

   A. The mistake is not participating in prevention programs, such as getting flu and other shots and checkups

   B. Prevention initiatives are often free and are always cheap compared with treatments. Take advantage of all opportunities to get compliments about how well you're doing, and to learn if there are issues to watch more closely.

10. Asking for help.

   A. The mistake is not asking for it when needed.

   B. Demonstrate that you are not shy, senile or backward. Be a human dynamo in the doctor's office, asking whatever questions come to mind and offering a bit of advice to the doctor as to how he or she might benefit from some wellness initiative you have found particularly appealing! There is no law that says you can't give the doctor a bit of free advice just because he/she is getting paid to give advice (and/or treatment) to you.

That's it—a positive spin. A cheerful outlook that looks on the bright side and accomplishes the same objectives as telling some old guy or gal, like you or me, that he/she is doing ten things wrong!

I respect folks who volunteer. Tens of thousands of good people, many retired, do good work in countless causes and ask little or nothing in return, except perhaps a bit of joy in being of service. However, sometimes volunteer labor does more harm than good, for the volunteer, or the cause, or both. As a cheerfully skeptical person, I have reservations about volunteering and I'll tell you why.

My advice: Volunteer for any of a number of good reasons, but also be aware of the possible downsides. Be a volunteer, not a martyr or hopeful candidate for sainthood or something. Be certain you are not eliminating a paying job—an army of retired and other good-hearted folks who just want to stay engaged could fill a post that someone else who needs a paying job would otherwise have. Consider that a job worth doing is worth getting paid for. Sometimes volunteers relieve government or its agents of responsibility to care for the needy or carry out other appropriate functions. Also, underlying social problems can be made to appear more manageable by the presence of volunteers, thus delaying necessary, comprehensive solutions. Other times, volunteers are exploited. In many volunteer situations, some folks ARE being paid. Why not you?

If YOU plan to volunteer, set some standards. Work on your terms, not someone else's. Seniors are often easy marks for exploitation. Have none of that. Make sure you enjoy or otherwise feel good about whatever you are doing and don't overdo it to the point that it runs you down. Make sure your volunteering does not delay longer-term, systemic reforms because of the ameliorative short-term benefits of your service. No point in making others dependent on your services, since you (and other volunteers) won't always be around. Be a good

TIP

34

To Be or Not To Be— A Volunteer

Other things being the same, it's usually best if they pay you for it

example to others if you do volunteer by staying focused on healthy lifestyle practices, especially if others seem stressed or in need of lifestyle reforms.

My friend Sandy Scott, a polymath with whom I share many interests (wellness lifestyle dynamics, cycling, running, philosophy and an admiration for our beautiful wives and other women, to note just a few), expressed reservations about this tip. (Perhaps "reservations" is not the precise, exact term that applies here. He basically thinks my notions about volunteering suck.) For the benefit of others who might share all or parts of Sandy's points of view about volunteering, I'll quote and then briefly comment on a few of his demurrers:

"If I decide to volunteer my services, I cannot burden myself with the woes of the world (am I taking a potential job from someone else, etc.)."

I agree with Sandy on this. If someone wants to volunteer, I say, "Go for it." My comments were intended only as points of view to consider.

"If I volunteer for some under-funded animal shelter, I guess I can insist on a salary knowing that there will be less money available to assist the animals with food, shelter and being placed in good homes. Is the fact that the director gets paid (to support his family) reason for me to demand my share of the pie—especially when my net worth is rather high? Methinks not. The good thing about volunteering is that you always work on your terms in that you are free to leave a microsecond subsequent to said terms being compromised by those to whom you volunteer your services."

Once again, I agree. It seems my writing leads sensible people to think I don't like animals! Or, that I somehow assume that once you volunteer, you're stuck in that role forevermore. I'll put it this way: Having a sound awareness of the situation in which you become involved is a good idea for everybody.

"I fear complicating everything we do with new rules (get paid, don't compromise, etc., etc.)."

Like Sandy, I would not want to have to deal with a lot if any "rules," especially when I'm a volunteer. These tips are offered as suggested considerations if one is so disposed to ponder any of them. Definitely not rules. (On the other hand, if I thought I could get away with setting down a few commandments, well, that would be tempting!)

"Let me answer your question, 'If a job's worth doing, why shouldn't you be paid for doing it?' Because you feel so passionately about something that you are willing to donate your valuable time and talent to make something better by your presence. I suppose we can put a value on everything we do, but there are more important ways to measure something than in terms of how much money an endeavor returns to you."

This may come as a surprise but the fact is I agree. Wholeheartedly.

A pity I did not engage Sandy as my co-author on this book project when I began taking notes on tips for aging under the influence 69 years ago. Everything I wrote subject to misinterpretation due to my wild and crazy writing style would be impossible to misconstrue, incapable of not being persuasive and absolutely not ridiculous, mean-spirited or simply jejune. Maybe.

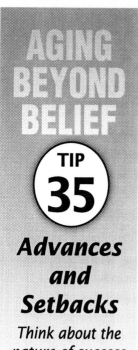

AGING BEYOND BELIEF

TIP 35

Advances and Setbacks

Think about the nature of success and failure, especially yours

*E*verybody succeeds and fails, regularly. Many of our failures in life are not such a big deal; and some, seen as big deals, turn out not to have been so momentous, after all. The same is true for our successes. Often, both lead to new directions, insights and opportunities.

But, let's focus on failure for a while. Some people, perhaps most, fail grievously, and do so often and consistently. Failures can be catastrophic, unrecoverable and disabling. For many in the throes of failure, things are never good again, and life spirals downward into the abyss. Napoleon Hill wrote, "Life's greatest tragedy consists of men and women who earnestly try and fail! The tragedy lies in the overwhelmingly large majority of people who fail, as compared to the few who succeed. I have had the privilege of analyzing several thousand men and women, 98% of whom were classed as 'failures.'" There is something radically wrong with a civilization, and a system of education, which permits 98% of the people to go through life as failures." (*Think and Grow Rich!: The Original Version, Restored and Revised,* Ross Cornwell, 2004).

If Hill's assessment is more or less accurate, and semantics plays a big role in this assessment, then surely there is something radically wrong with our education system, if not our civilization. If we set high standards for such an assessment, then Hill is probably right. That is, if we take account of the awesome knowledge and tools at our disposal today relative to what existed throughout human history, our own time should be a utopian millennium, considering the criterion of our potentials. Instead, look what we have: wars, famines, environmental degradation, ignorance and superstition on massive scales and more perturbations of all kinds. Maybe Hill was an optimist!

But, let's get personal. Where would you put yourself on an imaginary continuum between success and failure?

Success_____x_____Failure

+10   neutral   -10

No matter where you placed the mark today, know that it can change tomorrow—or next year, especially if your notions of success or failure change.

A sense of personal success, at some level, seems a requisite for AUI of a wellness lifestyle. That is, IF aging is to encompass human happiness, morality and a meaningful, good life. A mindset that elevates science and reason, a conscious appreciation of ethics, art, beauty and conscience seems to me a vital element of a worthy standard of success, one that is at least as consequential as material comforts and acquisitions.

Charles Dickens, in his 1849 classic autobiographical classic, *David Copperfield*, offered this immortal line on success or failure (first sentence of the book): "Whether I shall turn out to be the hero of my own life, or whether that station will be held by anybody else, these pages must show."

You write the pages of your failures and successes daily, not only in what you do (or fail to do) but in how you respond to events and circumstances. Here are a few tips for boosting chances of making the most of your successes and the least of your failures.

- You are not a failure if you don't feel like or consider yourself one. Be kind—give yourself a boost—a vote of confidence. Be generous and kind-hearted toward your own contributions. After all, if YOUR grandfather had been a US Senator and your dad president and you grew up amidst privilege, you probably could have been president, too. If so, it's likely you would have been a greater success than "the Decider," whose failure Ann Richard's once explained as follows: "Poor George. He can't help it—he was born with a silver foot in his mouth."

- Always be mindful of the fact that life is intrinsically unfair and unjust, that there is no escape from pains and sorrows, gloom and doom, that you face life alone and change alters everything—and then you die. This will ensure that every failure (and success) remains in perspective.

- You are responsible. Don't waste time and energy on excuses, blaming or explaining.

- Live honestly, with integrity and, as the Buddha is credited with teaching, by "immersing yourself in the river of life."

- Aging is a test of how well you can adjust to change processes of personal evolution over time. Growing older is a test for all social classes, all races and all people.

What, then, are realistic, objective measures of success and failure? Such measures will always be somewhat subjective and personal, but not entirely. After all, most of us don't want Ted Bundy, OJ Simpson, Tom DeLay or countless other infamous characters widely viewed as successful, no matter how they choose (and manage) to think of themselves. This matter of objective success measures deserves more attention that I can give it here, or elsewhere, but we do need some consensus. How can we better understand those who contribute value to society, however unheralded? Who amongst us helps others improve, move in a direction of positive social and other advances consistent with common decencies?

Also, it might be nice if society could offer more compassionate and effective supports to people who are failing. While I would not want to inhibit individualism and freedom, it would be consistent with AUI if more ways could be found to help greater numbers of people everywhere to succeed in free and open societies.

In summary, it seems an AUI of a wellness lifestyle outlook entails a view that success is relative. We can set modest standards and then try to realize and perhaps exceed them. Doing so might help us feel successful, for a while. Ultimately, we're all the same—dead.

So, look on the bright side, while you can. Make a lot of most days, build up your muscle mass with exercise and select a sensible diet. Seek peace and harmony. Give something back and, if it's not too much of a bother—try to be of some service. Find ways to participate in one or more communities where you feel supported, appreciated and valued. Learn and practice self-management skills. Do half of these things and you should be a success. Do most of them and consider a run for higher office—we need you, desperately.

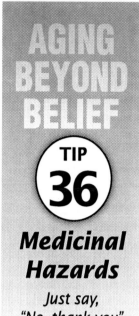

AGING BEYOND BELIEF

TIP
36

Medicinal Hazards

*Just say,
"No, thank you"
as often as possible
to drug-taking
opportunities*

*T*hirty years ago, I wrote, in "High Level Wellness: An Alternative to Doctors, Drugs and Disease," that "no medicine is good medicine, as a bendable rule." Well, it seems many folks have been bending the rule, if indeed they paid any attention to it in the first place. Would you believe that a quarter of adult Americans—and more than 40% of those of us 65 or older, take five or more medicines a week? Hard to imagine, but we do. Doctors worry that one medication cancels another, or worse, interacts with others, sometimes with dire consequences. So, the fewer you use, the better off you are, other things being the same.

Interactions between drugs are always a potential hazard, and problems occur when one inhibits the enzymes needed to clear another from the body. This can lead to a build-up of substances, which lead to toxic side-effects or a drug overdose. So, if you are taking drugs now, ask your doctor how you might cut back—and do some independent research on your own. Be particularly careful where alcohol is included in the mix. Did you know that abuse is epidemic among older adults? Evidently, many seniors drink too much because they are bored, or to ease anxiety or depression or as a sleep aid. Come to think of it, isn't this why everybody drinks? With seniors, however, the behavior is more likely to go unnoticed. (The older drinkers are less likely to be operating heavy equipment, quarterbacking an NFL team, flying airplanes or doing brain surgery.)

Furthermore, some believe older folks have few pleasures remaining and should be allowed to drink as they like. Well, of course EVERYONE should be allowed to drink him or herself into a stupor, if that's what he/she wants, but let's be as creative as possible in providing more healthful, attractive and joyous alternatives to our friends so tempted, whether young or old.

Abusive drinking amongst older folks, which accounts for a significant but unknown percentage of drug interaction problems, is often associated with falls, gastrointestinal disorders, stroke, cancer and varied other chronic conditions; according to a study by Wendy Adams and co-researchers.

A few years ago (1989), a study published in the *Journal of the American Medical Association*, (270; 1993) showed the rate of alcohol-related hospitalizations for Medicare beneficiaries was 54.7 per 10,000 men and 14.8 per 10,000 women. Alcohol-related hospital charges billed to Medicare totaled more than $233 million.

Basically, the drugs are new, the patients taking them in quantities are mostly old, but the problem is the same now as it was in 1977 when I wrote, "no medicine is good medicine, as a bendable rule." People expect too much of drugs and too little of themselves. An exercise prescription is a preferred alternative to many of the expensive meds being taken to excess and in combination with others.

There is a grassroots campaign that seeks to promote health and boost the quality of life for Americans. It is called "Just Say Know To Drugs." It was created to discourage people from overusing drugs. The "Just Say Know" (JSK) campaign focuses on what parents should know about drugs too readily made available to their children, as well as their own use of drugs. The year-round JSK campaign tries to motivate people to look closely at prescription medications—and to explore ways to cut back or eliminate meds entirely. The goal at first was to motivate a million Americans to ask their doctors: "What am I really putting into my body—and what are the alternatives?" JSK wants parents to audit their medicine cabinet and explore, with medical providers, the nature of what they put into their own and their children's bodies. For more on JSK, call 212-861-7400, email to JSK at info@psychtruth.org or visit the campaign website—www.psychtruth.org/Justsayknow.htm

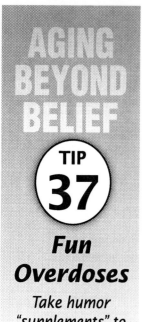

AGING BEYOND BELIEF

TIP 37

Fun Overdoses

Take humor "supplements" to mitigate joint aches and pains—and for other benefits, as well

*D*o your joints ache? Well, if you are in your 50s or older and you have not eaten well for years and you are not fit, what do you expect? You're lucky to be alive. Dr. Don (i.e., yours truly) recommends long walks for fitness and weight loss, if necessary. My AUI RDA (recommended daily allowance) or prescription—23 units of belly laughs daily—minimum! Also, lots of good deeds and a big cutback on the painkillers. Your pain killer meds might be popular brand meds (e.g., Celebrex and Vioxx), but also count in this category such things as aspirin and booze (not that your doctor prescribed the latter). My prescription is free, whereas the meds are not, so you will save money on my "no medicine is good medicine" approach and have more fun, even if your joints still hurt. Humor will get your mind off the aches, for a while. Then, look for some more—humor, that is.

Another benefit of an AUI wellness approach to joint pain is you will suffer less stomach upset and bleeding, two common side effects of the leading brand name drugs. No need to discuss your humor-based self-treatment program with your doctor, but do inform your caregivers about medications or other treatments you are taking. This applies also to unconventional treatments, in the event you are into New Age or "alternative" experiments (not recommended). Most medical centers are equipped with computer resources that permit tracking problems associated with specific drug combinations. However, unless you inform the health care professional, he/she won't know what drug interactions to investigate.

Some of the biggest interaction problems arise with over-the-counter remedies that are self-prescribed, not prescription drugs. These include not just the usual meds but also herbal supplements and vitamins. It is estimated that 16% of people using a prescription medication also take one or more herbal supplements or vitamins. Popular among these add-ons are antacids, calcium supplements and St. John's Wort. Doctors who prescribe a remedy are often unaware of other stuff being ingested and thus are unable to warn of adverse consequences.

Now you know the problem with interactions. Now you know to be alert. Now you know why I still favor no medicine as a bendable rule. Whatever your age, live well and cheerfully, find fun things to do and look on the bright side of life, even if it's a struggle to do so.

Don't overlook a bit of merriment in the dark humor associated with the vagaries of growing older. Golda Meir said, "It is not a sin to be seventy but it is also no joke." (*Memoirs: My Life*) Seek a heightened sense of the light side of things—and make yourself the punch line. For example, tell people why you are too old to go trick or treating on Halloween: "I'd have to get another kid to chew the candy for me!" Or, "I'd be afraid that when someone dropped a candy bar in my bag, I'd lose my balance and fall over."

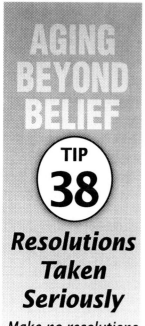

AGING BEYOND BELIEF

TIP 38

Resolutions Taken Seriously

Make no resolutions for the coming New Year—resolutions are too important for that!

*T*he New Year is celebrated for many things, but an occasion for effective resolutions is definitely not one of them. Resolutions made on January 1st are rarely realized. What's more, those who make such resolutions are almost always ill prepared for such an important activity. Either they don't organize the resolution process sufficiently or they don't take it earnestly enough! I wish to suggest a new custom: more frequent celebrations of the new and the old year, throughout the year. Why wait for a single day of merriment and celebration? If anything, let the real New Year's Day be a day to give resolution-making a rest.

Making resolutions at the start of the year tends to get rushed, given all the football games on TV, not to mention the headaches many suffer from excesses on New Year's Eve! However, The shaping of daily resolutions, especially if they invite a bit of stocktaking and reflection upon your good fortune and opportunities, is worth doing. Why not celebrate the occasion of new days every morning, in a positive and fun, ritual manner? It can be done with the whole family, if you have a whole family, or parts thereof.

The celebration could be a bit different each day, or have features everyone seems to enjoy. Examples might be, "Today I will give everyone who has the good fortune to encounter me my best smile," or, "Today I will be positive to an amazing degree," or "I shall take responsibility for my actions and results throughout the day."

Well, I'm sure you can dream up better examples. I doubt you will have any difficulty recognizing fortunate realities that richly warrant a little rejoicing of a ritual nature each day.

A wellness lifestyle requires discipline, responsibility, perspective and a mindset focused on excellence. While it is worth taking seriously, at the same time you don't need to be overly resolute or grim about it.

A wellness lifestyle is good for you. It is invigorating and entails limitless advantages for your family, your mate, significant others, friends, co-workers, and your country and the world. So, resolve to be a little bit better each day.

After all, AUI of a wellness lifestyle is not about health as much as it is about life—a life challenging, satisfying and meaningful. Celebrate being on track, approaching your potentials, making the most of genetic and other possibilities. Surely a resolution of some kind, just a momentary reflection on your commitment to artful living, will add to the day.

That's why you can with impunity forego the once-a-year, meaningless resolutions in favor of toasting your good fortune daily while looking on the bright side of life.

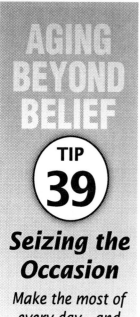

AGING BEYOND BELIEF

TIP 39

Seizing the Occasion

Make the most of every day—and go into positive action during the occasional crisis or challenge

*L*ife is populated with many crises and challenges, some of which are predictable, some not. The latter include life changes (e.g., hot flashes) and other aspects of aging. AUI promotes the perspective that it's better to do more than cope. With a self-responsibility model, you are more likely to regroup, then set to work seeking to THRIVE, not just adapt. Survival is good, survival is essential, but a predisposition to seize the day and transcend the ordinary is much better.

This attitude towards challenges/adaptations enables new levels of excellence and delight. Examples are "lose a job, seek a better profession; suffer an illness, overcome it or find ways to adapt to it."

Mark Twain knew of our too-human tendency to shy away from responsibility, as seen in this from *The Gilded Age*: "No one is willing to acknowledge a fault in himself when a more agreeable motive can be found for the estrangement of his acquaintances." Ask yourself, in the spirit of Joseph Heller's Yossarian, "Who is the enemy?" Yossarian's timeless answer in *Catch 22* was "the enemy is anybody who shoots at you—and anybody who sends you out to be shot at." So, don't settle for normalcy, also known as mediocrity. The enemy or obstacle is anybody, or anything, that puts you in harm's way. Don't be your own enemy.

Maybe, as the late Robert F. Allen advised, it is the unseen cultures, norms, customs, and rituals you adopted, little by little, over time with no deliberation or study, that is the enemy of being your best. "What is the answer?" you might wonder? Well, I don't know, it all depends on lots of things. But, I recall Woody Allen once said, "Love is the answer, but while you are waiting for the answer sex raises some pretty good questions."

As Andrew Marvell (1620-1678) put it, in "To His Coy Mistress:"

> But at my back I always hear
> Time's winged chariot drawing near;
> And yonder all before us lie
> Deserts of vast eternity.

One of the many motivators for and rewards of consciously choosing positive health habits is to slow the aging process. You want to achieve a compression of morbidity, reducing the period of time of infirmities. According a government report entitled "Healthy People," the impressive 76-plus years of life expectancy is encumbered by an average of 11.7 years of disability.

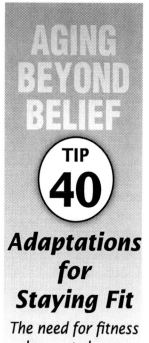

Adaptations for Staying Fit

The need for fitness does not change with age, but how to sustain it does

*T*he need for fitness does not change with age, but how to sustain fitness does. While I do not recommend shuffleboard, water aerobics or other stereotyped exercises for anyone as old as me or even close to my advanced age (except for fun, if that's your idea of a good time), I do advise exercising good sense, as well as the other muscle groups. No matter how fit you are, no matter how fast or how accomplished, the reality is that your ability to absorb, deliver and transport oxygen and everything else diminishes over time. Yesteryear's most highly engineered, fine-tuned, state-of-the-art thermodynamic engine needs to be red-lined a bit less often when the chassis qualifies for antique license plates.

Some of the most important things to consider as the years pile up are:

- Moderate your goals. Age group competitions are wonderful for runners, triathletes, swimmers, bikers and other endurance sport competitors. You don't have to run, swim, bike and so on as fast as you did ten years ago, which physiologically of course you simply can't—you just have to do such things faster than your peers, or age cohorts. As you get really, really old, like me, you can do this in John Travolta fashion—by staying alive, staying alive—and showing up!

- Bear more weights, not the meaningless burdens of stresses and worries. Even if you exercise daily with long, brisk walks or otherwise engage in glorious endurance exercises, like swimming, racquet sports, dancing or biking regularly in a strenuous fashion, you need resistance training two or three times a week. So, pump iron—or something. Weight-bearing exercise is activity supported by your skeleton. It will help maintain a leaner muscle mass, keep your metabolism high and also retain calcium. So, as Lance Armstrong's coach Chris Carmichael advises, "bone up on calcium right now." (*5 Essentials For A Winning Life*, Rodale Press, 2007, p. 109).

- Remind yourself that timing is everything. If you are a competitor, pick your battles. I used to run two, sometimes three road races in one weekend. Now I pick one or two a month—and some of my friends say that is way too much. Recovery takes longer later in life than in the early years. While this is common sense, it's astonishing how many experienced older athletes who should know better (and probably do) ignore the reality of it—and get injured as a result. I include myself in this category, but I'm working on it. Learn the easy way, from the mistakes of others. Pace yourself and choose the times when strenuous efforts are most desirable—and rest sufficiently before and after your heroics.

- Add quickness, timing, agility and/or balance-reliant activities now and then to your exercise routines. Reflexes wane with age, pretty much as does everything else. However, agility and the rest can be saved or restored in good measure with drills and routines that revitalize neural pathways between your brain and your muscles. Use diverse moves and motions and you will find you can go one way or another more cohesively, in a better-integrated fashion. This can enable you to take improved evasive action if some kid suddenly hurtles down the street in your direction on a skateboard, or if you find yourself, as I did, playing on a trampoline with your grandchildren.

If there is one thing that vexes me (and there are several, actually), it's being outmaneuvered by my granddaughter and grandson, both two years of age. It's hard to retain one's panache if, due to neglected agility, one is out "jumpy jumped" by people wearing diapers.

TIP
41

Artful
Living

If you insist on getting older, do it with panache, verve, style, and perspective

*T*he latter involves not worrying about how LONG you live, but focusing instead on how to have the most fun WHILE you live. Don't overlook exceptional health, either. Sure, you can and will get older, but maybe not a lot older. Look at it this way. Charlie Chaplin is dead, Adolf Hitler is dead and now Maria Esther de Capovilla is dead, too. Maria Esther had little in common with the beloved "little tramp" movie director or the infamous Nazi dictator, except for one thing—they were all born in 1889. At the time of her demise a month before a birthday party planned in her honor, Maria Esther was recognized as the oldest living person on earth at 116 years old. Word from Guayaquil, Ecuador where she lived and died is that the party was held anyway. No doubt her memory was fondly toasted by all in attendance, merrily eating cake and ice cream, thereby shortening their own lifespans.

It's not likely Maria Esther ever set a goal of living to 116, at least not before she reached 115. I don't think you should set such a goal, either, because you can't control enough of the operant variables, no matter how much you exercise, eat right and otherwise live a near-perfect lifestyle in an ideal climate with an adoring support system.

But you can get older, and surely will, for a while. If you are reasonably well now, you can do better than most by accepting the fact that about 77 years might be a possibility. That's the average life expectancy. But, it depends. It depends on a lot of things, mainly genetics and chance. Set sensible expectations, and be careful that your money and health don't expire before you do. Except for some obvious things (vigorous daily exercise, good nutrition, not worrying too much, finding meaning, laughing a lot, refraining from running with scissors and so on), you really can't do much to boost longevity. There's no shortage of vitamin sales people hawking resveratrol or the latest fad ingredient and other variations of snake oil who will try to persuade you otherwise. Basically, genetics and chance are the keys, and those are not subject to a lot of manipulation. The average life expectancy is 77. It is not the average life expectancy for people who have already made it to adulthood, much less 50 or 60. For such folks, already aging (hopefully under the influence of you-know-what), life expectancy is greater than 77.

So, live it up a bit or, better yet, a lot—today, while you're still a kid, at least compared with Maria Esther de Capovilla.

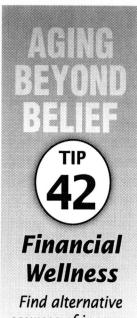

Financial Wellness

Find alternative sources of income, so as not to depend on social security

*N*othing wrong with Social Security, mind you, but I don't think it's going to be around much longer, at least not in its present somewhat generous form. Before explaining why, a little perspective seems in order.

Do you have any idea what life expectancy was throughout almost all of human history? Only 27 years. Most of our distant and not so distant ancestors died very young. The causes of death were infections, disease, hunger, homicide/war and non-human predators. Up until the middle of the 18th century, life was grim by our standards for all but a few. People did not have the luxury of pondering the meaning of life; I doubt much attention was given to reflecting upon the nature of wellness lifestyles. The primary focus was survival, shelter, strategies for securing the next meal and perhaps planning a conquest now and then, or how to defend against one.

Life got better, and a bit longer (by about 30 years), for the proverbial masses around the turn of the last century, thanks to better nutrition and an assortment of public health advances, particularly antibiotics, sanitation measures that controlled air and water borne diseases, immunizations and a modicum of health education.

Today we have life expectancy (at birth) of 77 or more, and the prospect of living much longer. How MUCH longer? One-zero-zero (100) is a reasonable possibility—something our ancestors would hardly have imagined. In fact, living to 100 could soon be commonplace.

Unfortunately, extended life spans for most will bring a special set of problems. One fearsome trend already well recognized is that birth rates will soon be insufficient to ensure the usual generational subsidy of the aged. In a few years, there will be too few young people paying into social plans that enable old workers to live in a fashion to which generations before them became accustomed. Consider that just three years ago, the U.S. population age 65 and older was 35.6 million. A scant quarter century from now, it will be twice that. Everyone over 100 years of age living in America today could fit in one of the stadiums hosting a New Year's Day bowl game. However, by the middle of this century, assuming each stadium capacity remains at about 85,000 seats, it will take 15 of them to hold all the centenarians expected at that time.

Here is a partial summary of trends that will require changes in Social Security (SS), Medicare and other safety-net traditions that have been in place for more than half a century.

- When SS was set up after the Depression years in 1935, benefits kicked in at the benchmark age of 65. Why 65? Because life expectancy at the time was 61. If SS were established today using the same parameter, benefits would be set at age 81 or 82! No need for actuarial tables to figure out real quickly that current SS finance projections would be much rosier under this scenario.

- At current trend rates, SS annual deficits will commence in 2018; bankruptcy will follow in 2042. The outlook for Medicare is even grimmer—that program goes broke by 2020.

- The necessary changes to keep SS and Medicare sound are beyond the integrity level of current politicians. To protect the solvency of the programs, benefits must be restricted and/or the eligibility age must be raised. As described by Sylvester J. Schieber and John B. Shoven in The Real Deal: The History and Future of Social Security, "elected officials have a tendency to focus on downstream issues within the context of two-year election cycles."

Some experts suggest less focus on the repair of social programs and more on rethinking retirement, suggesting that it makes little sense to retire at 65 if we live to 95. Fortunately, this change is underway, as noted recently when 70 percent of 45-year olds polled by the AARP reported plans to work well past retirement age. Why? Economic worries, in particular the astronomical cost of "health" insurance. Good thinking, boys and girls.

According to scholars at the Lifespan Development Laboratory at Stanford, if you passed age 30, you're already dying. "That's when cell death begins to outstrip cell replacement," the lab director has declared. Fortunately, there are enough reserves in most of our organs to keep us going all the way to 100 or so, provided our genes are favorable, we have good fortune (avoid random acts of disaster) and IF we've looked after ourselves sufficiently. Yet, how many Americans have been doing the latter? The worst of all scenarios is not only dramatic increases in the elderly population and reductions in the number of working young, but aged populations who are physical wrecks in need of expensive health care! It gets worse—that needed care must be obtained from a dysfunctional medical system. That means the cost of even low quality government entitlement and charity programs, drugs, medical procedures, warehousing and all the rest will prove economically disastrous or, more likely, such supports will not be available at all. In that case, the infirm aged will be on their own under conditions akin to those endured by soldiers in Napoleon's Grande Army trying to make their way home from Moscow during the winter of 1812. In other words, a grim scenario.

The moral of this tip is pretty simple: Shape up or ship out—IF you know what's good for you. I know you do. Bottom line—stay well and accumulate lots of money. Or, marry a rich person, as I did.

Make a conscious choice to safeguard your self-respect and honor the real celebrity, the one who matters most—yourself. Consider ignoring or at least not taking seriously strangers with familiar names—just because they are familiar. Safeguard your dignity. Reassess how you choose to perceive and respond to society's so-called celebrities. There is a lot of celebrity worship in most cultures, including ours. People unconsciously allow themselves to be taken in by the forces that profit from this chicanery, those who foist upon us marketing gimmicks, PR flacks and other opinion manipulators. Consequently, citizens become smitten by the rich and famous, including the infamous. I'm sure you can think of examples, as I can but I won't mention here on advice from my attorneys!

Celebrities, Self-Esteem, and Mental Health

No, I don't want your autograph

Symptoms of being overly impressed by others, with consequent inattention to your own merits as one (at least) equally deserving of regard and respect, include:

- A tendency to buy fan magazines (scanning a mindless rag with insane headlines in a supermarket checkout doesn't count).

- Queuing for or otherwise seeking an autograph—unless you're planning to sell it, and that's not very nice.

- Reading vapid rags like "People" magazine.

- Screaming like a teenager in the presence of a "mighty personage."

Don't feel badly if you have fallen for this kind of celebrity trap—it's a cultural norm, something we do because we have seen everyone else doing it. Instead, wean yourself from it, henceforth. After all, unless you had been on guard against such a thing, you could not help acting like an unworthy servant to the rich and famous types— it's genetic as well as cultural. At least that's what recent scientific evidence seems to suggest. We are actually programmed to act like monkeys! Seriously!

A study dubbed "Monkeys Pay Per View," highlighted in the Wall Street Journal (February 11, 2005, B3.), describes the celebrity phenomenon amongst our ancestors. It seems monkeys are highly impressed by power and beauty. If there were a People Magazine for monkeys focused on the romances, troubles and gossip about powerful and beautiful simians, monkeys would buy it, according to neuroscientists at Duke University. The work of the Duke researchers explains why "monkeys will pay to see sexy photographs and images of high-status individuals within their own social groups." Sound familiar?

Experiments demonstrated that monkeys would surrender "hard-earned perks for a peek at pictures of the dominant leaders and nubile females in their troop." Much of this had to do with mate selection. Well, I have to admit, in my younger days, I myself might have surrendered a few hard-earned perks for pictures of nubile females in Playboy Magazine, though at the time I never imagined I was making a monkey of myself.

While all this fuss over celebrities is fine for jungle life, you are NOT going to find a mate reading gossip magazines about celebrities, most of whom would not give you the time of day, let alone an autograph! The study authors provide a conceptual framework for decision-making by humans as well as primates. The research shows, according to the lead author, that "people are willing to pay money to look at pictures of high-ranking human primates. When you fork out $3 for a celebrity gossip magazine, you're doing exactly what the monkeys are doing. The difference between the study and People Magazine is that the monkeys actually know the individuals in the picture."

So, don't act ape-like to establish a reputation or remind others and yourself that you exist. You don't have to be loud and rambunctious or, I might add, obnoxious or deferential. Your life is of more consequence to you than anything rumored to be happening to the stars featured in celebrity magazines. Perspective is everything—try to keep an outlook that is rationally attuned to your own best interests. I remember a visit to Australia a few years ago. My hosts treated me to a footy match (Aussie rules football) between the Hawks of Hawthorn and the Saints of St Kilda at the Telstra Dome in Melbourne. I did not have a clue what was happening on the field. However, it was great fun to watch the mayhem out there and marvel (in horror) at the passion of the fans. At game's end, clusters of female fans of the losing team (I can't recall who won or lost) in the top deck of the Dome were slumped in their chairs, weeping. I could not believe it. Then I realized that this is a worldwide phenomenon. The fans simply lacked a rational perspective. The same applies to those who emulate monkeys in other ways. It's a reflection of mindsets inconsistent with wellness lifestyles, in my opinion.

What do you think? Do you want to get over it, over the foolishness of "celebrity-itis?" It's a choice, after all. With more leisure time on our hands than young folks, seniors often fall into this trap. The biggest problem it entails might be that it implies that these characters are better than we are, more deserving of a fuss, which I don't think is true at all. Better they should be asking for YOUR autograph, since you and others who pay attention to them are the ones who make them famous in the first place. That's why I suspect you will want to safeguard your self-respect and honor the real celebrity. You know who that is—that handsome devil/gorgeous babe looking back at you when you brush your teeth. Give yourself an autograph and let someone else act like a monkey around the make-believe celebs.

I asked a number of people about this and received many interesting responses. One that added the most to my thinking on the matter and, more important, gave clarity to the tip, came from Bob Ludlow. "I have never had this celebrity-worship affliction. Long, long ago I came to the realization that I could learn best from the people I admired by READING their articles and books. What was so special about seeing them give a talk, unless of course the talk promised new, never-published information or insights? I also used to say I wouldn't walk across the street to see a celebrity or presidential candidate. There IS, as you imply, something intrinsically demeaning about being part of a large crowed gawking at a celeb. Now a live PERFORMANCE is quite a different thing, of course. I wouldn't even make any effort to meet and briefly talk to a celebrity—what's the bloody point? If I could sit down with someone famous and talk to him or her for an hour or so, that would be different. I would be interested in that. So no, I never got that gene. Isn't this part and parcel of the same tendency to give the president, or the pope, such exaggerated respect? I wouldn't feel the least bit intimidated by this president, obviously, or any president (or pope), for that matter. Like you said, I don't think they're better than I am. Chances are a lot of them have as much to learn from me as vice-versa. End of rant."

I'll explain what a DUI pill is in a moment. First, let me summarize the situation with respect to weight loss pills in general. Basically, even if the pharmaceutical companies are able to produce an effective weight loss pill, which is not something you want to hold your breadth awaiting, it will never deliver good health or improved fitness levels.

Too many people are already overly dependent upon pills to the point of neglecting healthy lifestyles, thinking they can get by with medications alone. Sir William Osler made note of this some time ago. He believed "the desire to take medicine is perhaps the greatest feature which distinguishes man from animals."

Weight Loss

When they invent a weight loss pill, give it a pass—unless it's a DUI pill

America needs something better for weight loss. Consider this excerpt from the Dietary Guidelines for Americans 2005: "In recent years, diabetes rates among people ages 30 to 39 rose by 70%. About 46.5 million adults in the United States smoke cigarettes, even though this single behavior will result in disability and premature death for half of them. More than 60% of American adults do not get enough physical activity, and more than 25% are not active at all." The Guidelines call for Americans to spend "60 minutes on physical activity on most days" and, most important for those with weight problems, "60 to 90 minutes of exercise to keep the weight off." Surprisingly, the US is not the only fat country.

A report out of Brussels by the International Obesity Task Force lists seven other European nations where the proportion of overweight or obese males is higher than here. Those achieving this dubious honor are Cyprus, the Czech Republic, Finland, Germany, Greece, Malta and Slovakia.

In America and elsewhere, no pill is likely to solve the obesity epidemic, even if it could be made widely available at affordable rates. What IS required is, as noted above, a vast change in public attitudes leading to healthier lifestyles, particularly regarding exercise. This means the evolution of a new norm of 90 minutes of exercise daily, plus (as the Guidelines advise), "consume fewer calories and more fruits, vegetables and whole grains. People should also drink more low-fat milk and eat less fat and salt."

I have a mind to manufacture a weight loss product and market it as a wellness wonder pill for permanent fitness. I could call it "Don's Ultimate Ingredient," or DUI. The chief side effects for someone who takes this DUI would be permanent weight loss, a more attractive body and more energy for life. DUI would NOT contain rimonabant or any other active ingredient, only a bit of water, sugar and a teeny weenie bit of coloring agent to make it look pretty. DUI would be cheap, maybe ten cents a pill and only one need be taken daily, but the pills would come with precise directions. It would have to be taken AS DIRECTED! Any failure to follow the AS DIRECTED prescription would guarantee failure. Here is how the AS DIRECTED notice would read, more or less: "Take one pill and exercise 90 minutes daily, consume fewer calories and eat more fruits, vegetables and whole grains." I might add, in a burst of originality, try to always look on the bright side of life.

On the other hand, IF scientists develop a safe and effective weight-loss pill (and that is a possibility, despite my skepticism stated above), those who do need to lose weight should take it, if they try, but for any reason do not get satisfactory results with my DUI.

If I ever get around to manufacturing DUI, I'll let you know about it. Meanwhile, do the AS DIRECTED part, and take comfort in the advice of Ben Franklin: "He's the best physician that knows the worthlessness of the most medicines." You don't need the pill, if unlike most Americans, you have good sense in lifestyle matters.

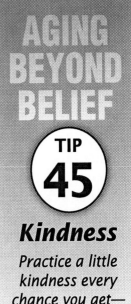

TIP

45

Kindness

Practice a little kindness every chance you get— and not just of a random nature

The Welsh writer Jan Morris recently urged British politicians to recognize kindness as a potent asset. You might want to do the same— it's not only good for others, but will benefit you, as well. Ms. Morris, author of dozens of artful travel books, observes that "few Britons go to church or chapel, most are probably agnostic if not decided unbelievers, and the rest are split into infinite sectarian divisibilities of faith." Simple kindness, on the other hand, needs "no theologians to explain it to us." ("Vote Kindness," *Wall Street Journal*, February 24, 2005, A14.)

What an amazing idea. Of course, another good reason to practice kindness is that it makes life better for everyone, not just British politicians. It embellishes the pleasures of life for all in a multitude of little ways and gratifies both purveyors and beneficiaries. Unlike religious paths, which "bore to death most of the electorate and antagonize the rest," an emphasis on kindness could impart a transcendental element to the amelioration of life's intractable difficulties. Indeed, Ms. Morris goes even further, suggesting kindness has such potential it could be used for commercial as well as political advantage. She suggests sample slogans, including, "Vote Tory: The Party of Kindness," and "Wisconsin Cheese: From The Land of Kindness." In summary, Ms. Morris believes there is "latent in the idea of kindness a great abstract weapon only waiting to be brandished: Grander than mere religion, far nobler than greed, more convincing than any political creed."

Well, Ms. Morris has distinguished company in a worldwide movement to promote this splendid virtue. About a decade ago, a "Small Kindness Movement" started in Japan. Soon, a conference was held, after which attendees fanned out across the globe to promote kindness. Many organizations devoted to kindness have been formed. Links to kindness organizations in twelve nations are available at www.worldkindness.org.sg

The best known of the kindness groups in America is "The Random Acts of Kindness Foundation." It exists as "a resource for people committed to spreading kindness." The Foundation's website offers materials such as "activity ideas, lesson plans, project plans, teacher's guides, project planning guides, publicity guides and workplace resources." All these resources are free. The basic idea is to inspire people to practice kindness and to "pass it on" to others. The Foundation's "kindness coordinators" assist others to incorporate kindness into thousands of schools and communities. The belief is that, "as people tap into their own generous human spirit and share kindness with one another, they discover for themselves the power of kindness to effect positive change. When kindness is expressed, healthy relationships are created, community connections are nourished and people are inspired to pass kindness on." Interestingly, the Foundation is privately funded—it accepts no donations, grants, or membership dues and, best of all, it has no religious, government or other affiliations. It truly appears to be an affirmative-action, equal kindness-opportunity organization.

Kindness is, of course, one of the common moral decencies widely shared, particularly by those for whom religions have no appeal. Paul Kurtz and many others view the common decencies as "the foundation of moral education" and high life quality in human communities. He sees personal integrity, trustworthiness and benevolence as moral standards for dealing with each other. Kindness is viewed as behaviors "manifesting goodwill and noble intentions toward other human beings." Kindness entails having a positive concern for other people. It makes us more sympathetic and compassionate. A practical example can be seen in this advice from Caitlin J. Noris in, "A Few Simple Rules for a Healthy Roommate Relationship," published in the Wall Street Journal Classroom Online Edition (December, 2003): "It is amazing how far kindness and respect will take you. Living in a small space with a stranger is sometimes awkward, but the tension can be eased by simply being polite." Just so.

I'll be kind at this point and stop belaboring the merits of kindness. Kindness is not hard to appreciate, though it is easy to overlook in the rush of daily life.

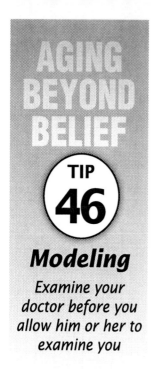

Modeling

Examine your doctor before you allow him or her to examine you

I created this short principle when I wrote my first book in the late 1970s, namely, *High Level Wellness: An Alternative to Doctors, Drugs and Disease* (Rodale, 1977). I still feel strongly about it today. There are three distinct kinds of information you should have about any doctor with whom you plan to do business.

The first deals with lifestyle. Does the doctor look after herself? Is it clear that she values personal responsibility, fitness, sensible nutrition and all the rest? Is this evident in the way she practices, and in the obvious message conveyed by her appearance? That is, does she look fit?

The second deals with basic competence—is the doctor well educated, up-to-speed with recent developments in her field and sufficiently knowledgeable to deserve your confidence and expectation of quality care? That is the first level of inquiry I recommend. Unfortunately, few patients, myself included, go to the trouble to establish a doctor's bona fides. We just assume that if a doctor has an office, patients, diplomas on the wall and wears the requisite white coat, she must have gone to medical school somewhere, is licensed to practice and, most critically, is competent. That, of course, is a leap of faith, but life is filled with daily leaps of faith, even for those of us who prefer science and reason.

The third level entails a check beyond medical skills. This is the level of character, judgment and human decency. It is also a leap of faith to assume that she is ethical. There are no checklists for this one, but you can get a sense by paying attention. Is she courteous, polite and empathetic? Is she sincere? Does she tell the truth, keep promises, avoid hypocrisy, honor agreements? Your doctor should be trustworthy, dependable and responsible. She should also be benevolent, fair, tolerant and ready and able to cooperate.

A few doctors might not take senior care as earnestly as you do. I suspect that some expect too little for older patients. If you suspect this for a micro-second, my advice is, "Fire your doctor!" You have every right to do this. If you do not like the way you are being treated, dismiss the hired help. Some seem not to consider that they can do this. We can and should, if warranted.

On the other hand some, maybe the vast majority of doctors are, like my general practitioner, just terrific and wonderful. Considering how hard they work and the pressures they face, good doctors are treasures and should be much appreciated.

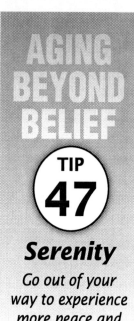

*T*here are untold ways you might do this. You could watch Oprah, drink alcohol, gorge on chocolate, avoid exercise and take dope. I don't recommend any of these things. Here are five things I DO recommend—for starters. I'm sure you can think of many more. Some of these are so important I have mentioned them before, in a different context, but they are all important enough to sneak in again, just to improve the chances you will adopt a few of them.

1. Get a grip. Adopt a reasonable perspective, such as this one: You are not even close to being the center of the universe. In fact, like me, you are more akin to a meaningless blob of nothing, in the grand scheme of things, if there WERE a grand scheme of things. Do you doubt this? If so, answer this: What is greater in number—grains of sand on beaches all over the Earth, or the number of comets, planets, and stars in the universe? The answer is comets, planets, and stars in the universe. There are between 200 to 400 billion stars in our galaxy alone (the Milky Way) and there are over a hundred billion galaxies, each with hundreds of billions of stars. If you are not breathing tomorrow at this time, it won't make that much difference, in the GRAND SCHEME of things. My point? Don't take yourself so seriously.

2. Make the most of the time you have, even though it doesn't matter that much. According to Vincent E. Parr ("The Art of Living: How To Feel Good Without Feeling Good About Yourself," *Free Inquiry Magazine*, Volume 25, Number 2), there are "8,760 hours, 525,600 minutes, or 31,536,000 seconds in one year ... In an average lifetime of 75.5 years, you will have 2,380,968,000, or approximately 2.4 billion, seconds, and that's it!" Use them well.

3. Save yourself a cavalcade of hardships—read and heed Ambrose Bierce's parting advice in the final edition of his "Town Crier" column in the *San Francisco Examiner*, March, 1872: "Be as decent as you can. Don't believe without evidence. Treat things divine with marked respect—and don't have anything to do with them. Do not trust humanity without collateral security; it will play you some scurvy trick. Remember that it hurts no one to be treated as an enemy entitled to respect until he shall prove himself a friend worthy of affection. Cultivate a taste for distasteful truths. And, finally, most important of all, endeavor to see things as they are, not as they ought to be." (*Ambrose Bierce: A Biography* by Richard O'Connor, Little, Brown and Company, 1967, NY, p. 83.)

4. Consider Walt Whitman's "Carpe Diem—Seize The Day," a line made famous in the movie "The Dead Poets Society" with Robin Williams, but forget trying to seize an entire day. Settle for being present fully in the moment, or "carpe momentum." As Dr. Parr suggests, "if you cannot enjoy the moment, right here, right now, then you probably cannot and won't enjoy life."

5. Find something you enjoy and, over time, try to get really good at it. Eventually, it will become one of the key aspects of your persona, if not your major passion. Hopefully, you will choose something positive that you will be proud of and it will give your life added meaning. Naturally, it will also lead to more peace and personal happiness, which is why the suggestion is included here. In *Catch-22*, Joseph Heller wrote: "Some men are born mediocre, some men achieve mediocrity and some men have mediocrity thrust upon them." I think we all are born into mediocrity, achieve plenty of it and have more of it thrust upon us. No matter—rise above it all in at least one aspect of life important to yourself.

Well, there you go. Five tips for more peace and personal happiness.

Hope some of them make sense and work out for you as part of your AUI mindset.

I'll suggest one in a moment. First, let me recount a story about how the motto I'm about to offer came to be. It's not likely true, but it's a fun story.

It seems there was, long ago, an Eastern monarch who was plagued by many worries and troubles. To deal with these vexations, he convened a counsel of alleged wise men. He asked them for fresh advice. He wanted a new motto, one that would give him wisdom in dealing with worries and troubles. However, the monarch set criteria for the motto that were quite formidable. He wanted a motto that would be brief, so brief it could be inscribed on a ring! This, he explained to the wise men, would make the motto available at all times. He added, "It must be appropriate to every situation, as useful in prosperity as in adversity. It must be a motto wise and true and eternally enduring, inspiring words by which a man could be guided all his life, in every circumstance, no matter what happens."

A Wellness Slogan

Consider adopting a really nifty motto

All the wise men thought and thought and finally came to the monarch with timeless words for every change or chance of fortune. They told the monarch the motto would fit every situation, good or bad. They said it contained words to lighten the heart and mind in every circumstance.

Are you ready for the motto the wise guys offered for engraving on the monarch's ring? I hope so. Here it is, the five-word motto that would fit nicely on the ruler's ring: "This, too, shall pass away."

My first reaction was, "pretty good advice," given the bizarre criteria for a motto laid down by the monarch. How the wise men did so well with no women involved is a bit of a mystery. But, a fine effort, nonetheless. That, at least, was my initial reaction.

However, after mulling it over for about 30 seconds, I had second thoughts. Did the monarch not know this already? Should this not be obvious to anyone, let alone so called wise guys? Did the monarch think some things would NOT pass away? What, for example, did he think would endure forever? His good looks, maybe? His monarchy? The favor of his women? Surely he knew that these and all things were temporal. Maybe he simply did not think about it, since he rewarded the wise men instead of hanging them.

If your tooth hurts or the weather is frightful or other vexations large or small tend to annoy, it helps, I suppose, to remind yourself that this, too, shall pass away. One does not need to be a monarch to benefit from this insight, and you need not have the insight engraved on a ring to remember it when the going gets tough.

*Y*our health status and life quality depend so much on a willingness to do more than is normal and customary to become and remain very fit and mentally healthy. You put a lot of energy into being well, healthy beyond the standard of just not being sick. That's why so many of the preceding tips deal with ambitious exercise, sound diet, having fun, finding added meaning and other such positive qualities. However, it is almost as important, if not equally so, to avoid doing things that set you back.

Shall I offer two obvious examples of habits that would set you back? Of course, I can't imagine you would do either of these things, but just for the record, I'll mention them anyway, since so many people (believe it or not!) still smoke and drink way too much alcohol. There, I just mentioned them.

TIP

49

Going Forward Without Falling Back

Don't sabotage your best efforts to live an AUI wellness lifestyle with pernicious missteps

It has been my experience over the course of 30 years promoting wellness lifestyles that doing the right thing (i.e., working at establishing and fine-tuning an artfully healthy, positive lifestyle) makes it much easier to refrain from risky habits. When you are feeling good about making progress, you attract positive attention and satisfying results. This motivates you to keep the momentum going forward, so wellness becomes a self-reinforcing choice.

Just to be on the safe side, however, consider the following nine preventive considerations. Some are medical in nature, others are unrelated to traditional health issues. All could affect your progress and results in AUI of a wellness lifestyle.

1. Medical checkups. Many checks are a good idea. However, being tested has its risks. Tests can be overdone. Read up on the options from varied sources and be discriminate about

145

consenting to testing. Just because something CAN be tested does not mean it ought to be.

2. Weight management. We gain about a pound a year after the mid-thirties. As described so well by the Red Queen in Lewis Carroll's *Alice in Wonderland*, weight control "takes all the running you can do, to keep in the same place. If you want to get somewhere else, you must run at least twice as fast as that!" Well, maybe not running, but brisk walking or some form of whole-body exercise is required to stay in the same weight place.

3. Hydration. Drinking a lot during endurance athletic events seems to have been overrated. In fact, some problems have been caused by drinking too much water and other fluids during marathons and such. The latest thinking suggests there is plenty of water in foods, soft drinks, coffee and tea, beer, wine, milk and so on. When you do drink water, consider that it need not be expensive bottled varieties that usually are no purer or otherwise superior to plain tap water.

4. Protect your skull. Always wear a helmet if you expose it by doing fun things that potentially put it in harm's way, such as riding a bicycle or motorcycle.

5. Be not a hermit. Get out there every day and connect with others. Allow plenty of time to socialize, including with friends and family.

6. Look after your largest organ! Your skin shields the rest of you beneath the surface from the environment. It is your main cooling system. Look after it. Safeguard your skin from the ill effects of our planet's star—wear protective clothing, use adequate sun block lotions and sprays and don't expose yourself to the sun in the middle of the day, if you can avoid doing so.

7. Don't live close to a toxic waste dump. Be aware of

occupational and environmental risks. A little investigatory snooping might reveal factors that can often be modified to lower risks at home, work and elsewhere.

8. If over 50, get shot. Keep your immunizations current, particularly booster shots every ten years for tetanus and diphtheria. Get flu and pneumonia vaccines annually.

9. Protect your smile—and ability to chew. Maintain good dental health. A cleaning every six months is advised by most dentists.

Wearing a helmet and following the other preventive steps will not make you fitter or healthier, as happens with most AUI strategies. However, by practicing these guides, you increase the odds that you will not suffer an avoidable decline in health and life quality. So while it's worth distinguishing between preventive and wellness-enhancing practices, both are important.

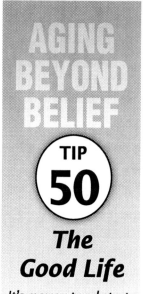

AGING
BEYOND
BELIEF

TIP

50

**The
Good Life**

*It's never too late to
discover, provided
you're breathing*

What does it mean to live a good life or
ideal life, to be a success? Mark Twain offered
this: "Good friends, good books and a sleepy
conscience: this is the ideal life." Perhaps,
but many have explored this question for
thousands of years. Libraries are filled with
books about the nature of a good and examined
life. A good life, success and all that surely
require values, purposes, morality—but which
values? Different groupings of people in
varied parts of the world have different, often
irreconcilable ideas along these lines. People
in the same country, town and even family
often have dramatically different values, as
we know from observing the machinations
of sanctimonious blowhards. (The latter are
political commentators with opinions at odds with mine.) Thus, one
possible response to the question, "What is the good life?" might
be, "it depends." It depends on whom you ask. (Edward Abbey
suggested, "The dog's life is a good life, for a dog.")

The choices we make, the habits we develop and the passions we
pursue are not even shaped and formed on a conscious basis. We
don't decide about the good life with all things considered, as
freethinking, rational adults. Instead, our basic "choices," habits
and lifestyles are shaped by the outside world, and set in our minds
long before we reach the age of reason. Only then can we make real
choices (or adjustments to early patterns) as conscious, rational and
freethinking adults. Of course, not everyone becomes such an adult.

Eventually, most of us get around to deliberately pondering the
nature of a good life, success and the rest. Some of us even find time
to think about and act upon ideas regarding the best kind of wellness
lifestyle. Always, however, we do so in accord with our cultures,
traditions and life experiences. Our lifestyles, therefore, are shaped

in accord with foundation societal value decisions, adopted and fine-tuned over time. The truly liberated adult will hone his or her philosophy and lifestyle, as new insights and experience suggest.

Now if you ask ME "What does it mean to live a good life, to be a success," I'm only too happy to oblige with a commentary. My response will be informed by my own cultures, traditions and life experiences—and supplemented by regular adult reflections on the matter.

A good life ensues from living in accord with common decencies. It is abetted by AUI of a wellness lifestyle that facilitates well-being, the realization of goals and the experience of affection and community. For more on all this, I recommend an editorial by philosopher Paul Kurtz entitled, "Two Competing Moralities: The Principles of Fairness Contra Gott Mit Uns!" (*Free Inquiry Magazine*, Vol. 24, # 4. Also available online at www.secularhumanism.org.)

For starters.

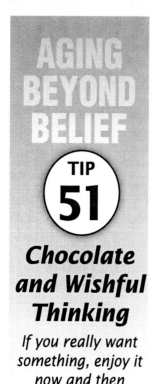

AGING BEYOND BELIEF

TIP 51

Chocolate and Wishful Thinking

If you really want something, enjoy it now and then

*T*ake chocolate, for example. Why ruin pleasure with guilt, self-loathing or pitiful attempts to justify something as good for you? Remember the song, "Enjoy yourself, it's later than you think?" (Music by Carl Sigman, lyrics by Herb Magidson, 1948.) It's true—even if you are not old, like me. Time's moving on so, chocoholics, get real. Enjoy your treats—just moderate the effects with an otherwise good diet and plenty of exercise. But please, don't latch on to those silly reports that chocolate in one form or another is good for you. That has to be a classic case of wishful thinking.

I had a dream the other night wherein my wife and I were in a crowded room filled entirely with addicts gathered for some kind of 12-step program. Suddenly, I was called upon. I stood, hesitant for a moment, and then realized the time had come to stop hiding my problem, to share my story, however shameful. With head high, I said, in a steady voice: "Hi. My name is Don, and my wife here is a chocoholic." Everyone was wonderfully supportive. "Hi Don," they cried joyfully in holistic unison. Yes, it was clear they could feel my pain and were with me all the way.

Although in almost every other regard she has more discipline over her lifestyle than I do, (and I'm a wellness guru, or so some of my less critical loyal followers think) where chocolate is involved, my dear wife is helpless. She knows better, but leaps to believe every half-baked study (one of which was based on a sample of thirteen people!) that seems to support the hope that cocoa beans are some kind of health food. A preposterous notion, in my opinion, demonstrating again the human tendency to believe what we want to be true. Recall the old expression, "If wishes were horses, then beggars would ride!" But, they are not and they do not. Or consider this bit of advice: Feel free to make fun of other people's idiosyncrasies while congratulating yourself on the lack of the same.

The claims by choco-maniacs and scientists who enjoy titillating them include the following:

- Chocolate is made from cocoa beans. Cocoa beans contain flavanols. Flavanols (some think) increase nitric oxide in the blood. More nitric oxide in the blood improves the function of blood vessels.

- Those who consume the equivalent of one-third of a chocolate bar daily have lower blood pressure —and a reduced risk of death. (This finding is based on a recent study of older Dutch men sponsored by the Netherlands Prevention Foundation).

Reality:

- Study participants who ate more cocoa products also were found to practice healthier lifestyles, which is probably what lowered their blood pressure. Chances are good that their lower blood pressures and risk of death developed DESPITE eating chocolate.

- These study subjects were also later found to have been lighter in weight and more oriented to eating nuts and seeds than those who munched on chocolates.

- The studies were done with male subjects; such data findings do not necessarily apply to females, and vice-versa.

- Eating too much chocolate can make you fat, which increases the risk of heart disease and high blood pressure. This can increase the difficulties of getting a date with a fit person.

- People do not just eat chocolate when they eat chocolate. As one Mayo Clinic doctor pointed out, "The problem is all the things people put chocolate with. The chocolate cakes, the chocolate ice cream." (Quoted in "Study Bolsters Chocolate's Tie To Better Health," *New York Times*, Page D6.)

Look—it could be true. Maybe chocolate is good beyond the favors of its flavonoid compounds. Maybe it makes you happier, improves your sexual functioning, improves your accuracy at tossing darts and brings you closer to God. Who knows? Nearly anything is at least theoretically possible, if not plausible. But, I wouldn't count on it. Live it up, eat chocolate moderately, if possible, indulge all kinds of other pleasures, but make time for serious daily exercise as well.

Let me end this heretical anti-chocolate rant with a learned reference to that great phrase-maker, Dr. Anonymous, who once told a chocolate fable: "This guy found a bottle in the ocean, and he opened it and out popped a genie, and he gave him three wishes. The guy wished for a million dollars, and poof! There was a million dollars. Then he wished for a convertible, and poof! There was a convertible. And then, he wished he could be irresistible to all women... poof! He turned into a box of chocolates." Mr. or Ms. Anonymous also is credited with this zinger: "There are four basic food groups: milk chocolate, dark chocolate, white chocolate, and chocolate truffles."

Finally, I'll leave you with this thought from Gina Hayes: "Make a list of important things to do today. At the top of your list, put 'eat chocolate.' Now, you'll get at least one thing done today."

Superstition

*Do your part
to combat
irrationality*

*D*on't be an easy mark for con artists and charlatans. Voltaire famously said, "The superstitious man is to the rogue what the slave is to the tyrant." Unscrupulous people and ridiculous customs can lead even sensible people like yourself to believe mind-numbing nonsense. The antidote is to prepare, in advance, to turn superstition back at every opportunity. Too many good folks put up with silly nonsense out of politeness, or a sense that confronting superstitions is just not worth the trouble. I think it is worth a bit of trouble. Speaking out against it and confronting it is a public service, a way of making a benevolent donation to the common good of the small segment of humanity you influence, however modestly. Besides, you can have a bit of fun being a skeptic about superstitions. My advice—reject all of it, in a good-natured way. Doing so will be a positive educational experience for others who benefit from your example. A superstition is a false belief based on ignorance. It is also defined as an irrational belief that future events are influenced by specific behaviors, without having a causal relationship. An historical example was the belief that certain incantations had to be uttered in certain ways to ensure that rains would come, crops would grow and everyone wouldn't starve; a popular modern superstition was to carry a rabbit's foot in order that bad luck would be avoided in the event a black cat crossed your path. These two examples are not wackier than most superstitions, yet superstitions continue to have a hold on vast numbers of people.

Consider Friday the 13th! Some folks still worry about bad luck due to a morbid, irrational fear of the conjunction of the sixth day of the week and the number 13. There is even a name for this fear—"par askevidekatriaphobia"—and 21 million people are said to have this condition, rumored to be THE most widespread of all superstitions. Irrationality, madness and total nonsense feed on forbearance. Speak up. Do your part to promote sanity by confronting madness.

The number of superstitions is unlimited, as anyone familiar with the diverse rituals of professional athletes before, during and after a game knows. Some of the most common superstitions (besides a rabbit's foot and black cats) involve walking under a ladder, breaking a mirror, something about a horseshoe, blowing out candles on a birthday cake, a chicken's wishbone—the list goes on, ad nauseam. While somewhat entertaining and usually harmless, superstitions are celebrations of irrationality. Such is nothing to celebrate—there is way too much of it in the world.

You can do your part to nibble away at such beliefs. Start with yourself—you might still harbor (unlikely, I'm sure) a superstition or two. Then reach out to friends and others to assist them to overcome unwise, irrational and injurious notions.

Not everyone has a personality profile that is conducive to speaking out. A different strategy from that I advise in this tip might be more appropriate for you. Briefly, you may do better NOT confronting superstitions and pseudoscientific claims. Let it all pass—just move along and keep the peace. There are other battles, perhaps, that you may want to wage, or none at all. It's sometimes a lot easier to finesse this kind of encounter, and then quickly change the topic. Doing so can avoid what may otherwise prove to be a tiresome discussion. If a friend or client believes in astrology, ESP, a living Elvis or that the South won the Civil War, for example, you may want to hold your tongue in order not to strain the relationship. It really depends on the nature and character of the relationship, as well as your sense of the pros and cons of full disclosure about your own worldview. Same with relatives or guests, especially if they are not likely to stay very long. For some folks, it's simply better to maintain a delicate, harmonious balance than to explore hot topics or sensitive controversies in the interest of full disclosure, the search for truth or whatever. It's a matter of style—your style and thus, your choice. Often, the price to pay for confronting nonsense is too great. It is good to ponder the best return on any investment, including your time and points of view. There are times, for some, when pleasant chit chat works nicely.

Robert Ingersoll, a famous Civil War-era rationalist and friend of Mark Twain, listed these characteristics of superstition over a century ago—and the guidelines still apply.

- To believe in spite of evidence or without evidence.

- To account for one mystery by another.

- To disregard the relation between cause and effect.

- To believe that mind created and controls matter.

- To believe in miracles, spells and charms, in dreams and prophecies.

- To believe in the supernatural.

Ingersoll viewed superstition as "the child of ignorance and the mother of misery." That's much too kind. Edmund Burke, the Irish orator, once said, "Superstition is the religion of weak minds." Personally, I think Burke came close but messed up the order of things. In any event, I'm guessing you don't want to attempt to AUI with a weak mind, so eradicate any lingering vestiges of superstition (not that you suffer any!) and help others do the same.

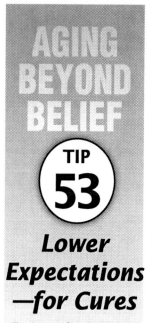

Lower Expectations —for Cures

Forget about magic bullets or other quick fixes for what ails you

*S*uppose you could take a pill that would make you slim, heart healthy AND enable you to overcome nasty addictions? Would you go for it?

I think most would, no questions asked, except maybe "How much?" or, "Is it covered by my insurance plan?"

Another important question might be, "Is it safe?" Other good questions would include:

- "What are the side effects?"

- "How does it work?"

- "What do the critics, if any, say about it?"

- "Are there other ways besides drugs to deal with my problems?"

The buzz that first brought this notion to mind was over an alleged wonder pill called "Acomplia." The company that sought approval for this multipurpose medicine made claims that sounded suspiciously like those you would hear for that elusive "magic bullet" that would cure everything with no adverse consequences. Somehow, the phrase "buyer beware" came to mind as I read the promotions for "Acomplia" (and the forecasts for the record sales and profits that would follow).

"Accomplia" was supposed to promote weight loss and smoking cessation, which in turn would enable cardiovascular benefits. Because of the American fat crisis, the profit potential of "Acomplia" seemed off the charts. Early estimates ran to at least $4 billion a year by 2010. Unfortunately for the manufacturer, the FDA turned down the company's first approval application due to concerns about adverse side effects. However, with additional studies, the OK might be granted, in time.

The processes by which "Acomplia" multitasks in the brain, fat cells, the liver, muscles and other body parts is not clear. This uncertainty, no doubt, gave the FDA pause. It is also a problem that distresses critics who warn of possible dangers. One drug scientist was quoted in news accounts: "Drugs that act on central nervous system receptors can do all kinds of odd stuff, and we most definitely do not know enough about brain chemistry to predict what those interesting surprises might be." (Scott Hensley, "Does a Drug for Many Ills Cause Too Many of Its Own?" Wall Street Journal, February 22, 2006.)

All drugs have risks; but a drug that creates a mass frenzy among willing drug takers looking for a fix is an escalation. Might there develop an "Acomplia" cult, with masses of folks creating another "fen-phen" craze, only later to learn that this fix causes problems worse than it was supposed to cure?

Some problems surfaced in the early tests. A number of users became nauseous, others anxious and depressed and some suffered sleep disturbances. All of which concerned many researchers about the long-term safety and effectiveness of the drug. Weight losses were not significant, either, and changes in addictive behaviors were less than remarkable.

"Acomplia" may, of course, turn out to be a wonder drug that does all that its backers hope and leads everyone to want to pursue wellness lifestyles and meaningful lives. But this is unlikely. The quest for magic bullets is marked with disappointments. The *Wall Street Journal* article cited above concluded on this sensible note: "Looking for risk-free drugs is a fool's errand, but it's equally foolish to ignore the fact that every benefit a medicine offers comes at a price. That price is paid over time in the side effects that patients suffer from medicines that may also help them. Makers of medicines with high promise, like Acomplia, must accept a high burden of proof as their price for admission to the market."

Be skeptical and take a wait and see attitude, not just toward

Accomplia but about all pills, magic-bullet or otherwise. Meanwhile, live well and wisely.

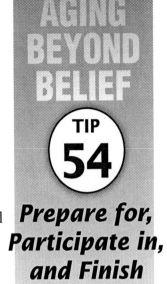

TIP

54

Prepare for, Participate in, and Finish a Triathalon

—and learn about managing change in the process

*I*f you declare yourself a triathlete, you may surprise your friends, annoy your enemies, impress yourself and amaze everyone else. Depending upon your age and situation, taking on this challenge might be a feat somewhere between impressive and remarkable. Of course, if you ARE a triathlete, experienced at this demanding sport, this tip won't be a big deal. You might consider another challenging physical feat that is a challenge for you that also requires preparation and offers an exciting finish.

The older you are, the more beneficial this tip will prove, when you pull it off. The rewards, that is, the pleasures, excitement and satisfactions of racing a three-sport event like a triathlon will flow from the experience itself, not the medal, trophy, plaque, ribbon or other symbol gained from winning or going faster than your peers. The latter can be fun, on occasions, but for us older folks, looking good and feeling terrific trumps everything else. What's more, the process is great for fine-tuning skills needed to manage change. These include making accommodations to obstacles, dealing creatively with setbacks, staying focused on the goal and celebrating achievements large and small.

While this tip might seem like a big deal or "a big ask," as the Aussies say, if you think "sprint" triathlon, the tip is quite doable, with a little bit of time and hard work. A sprint triathlon is but a quarter mile swim, a ten to fifteen mile bike and a 5K (3.1 mile) run. No big deal, if you do your homework (i.e., training).

Triathlon (swim, bike and run at varying distances) is one of the fastest growing sports worldwide. Showcased for the first time as an official event at the Sydney Olympics, triathlon originally came into public consciousness in the form of its most extreme manifestation,

159

the Hawaii Ironman Triathlon, thanks to broadcasts on ABC's Wide World of Sports. While good for the growth of the sport, the image of triathlon came to be that of an extreme sport, which at sensible distances it definitely is not. While the general public still thinks of triathlon as part epic quest, part insane hobby for exercise maniacs, it is in fact neither insane nor extreme for most who engage in it. Epic? Yes, a sprint tri could very well prove delightfully epic for you.

So, even if you are in your nineties or a centarian, consider the goal of preparing for and completing at least one sprint triathlon. You will get more fit in the process, build your confidence to attempt other advances, meet some wonderful people and be treated like a champion. Most important, you will feel like one—and isn't that reason enough to start swimming, biking and running? I think so.

USA Triathlon is the official governing body for the sport in America. If you accept this tip and begin your quest to complete a triathlon, you will come into contact with USAT. It had 80,000 members at the end of 2006. About half a million people did triathlons last year—many races were sold out months before the event took place. Don't wait too long to sign up for an event near you.

Naturally, there is much to learn if you decide to act on this tip. You want to discover, for example, the triathlon basics, such as training recommendations in each of the three sports, and you must learn about appropriate equipment, proper form and much more. But, all of these things can be and are enjoyable in their own right, if approached properly.

My first suggestion is to adopt a perspective of triathlon as metaphor for the larger challenges associated with managing change. This is a special value tip. In effect, two in one. Change is inevitable—maintaining the capacity to adapt throughout the years, especially those later in life is crucial to lifestyle success. The more confidence we feel about dealing with change, the more likely we are to be effective and prosper when change demands are encountered, both expected and unusual in nature. The multi-sport character of triathlon provides a dramatic and literal challenge of change in the form of two official "transitions" that are a part of every triathlon competition. These two transitions present the very same kinds of challenges you face on a regular basis in the human race. These challenges are often predictable and invite careful planning, just as is true for the athlete completing his first or thousandth triathlon.

When you set your sights on entering and completing a triathlon, you will want to plan for the necessary changes from the swim to the bike, and again from the bike to the run. These changes will take place in large spaces called "transition areas," where all the bikes, helmets, running and bike shoes, sunglasses and doping materials are stored. (Hahahaha—I'm kidding, of course. Just trying to keep you alert, as you are nearing the end of this book and may be in need of a little surprise now and then so as not to get depressed about so few tips left.) All these things (again, no doping materials—that was humor!) have been carefully arranged in advance of your arrival into the transition area during the actual race, so everything is where you put it, ready for your use at the appropriate time. Be cool about how you will manage the varied requirements in the transition area under time pressures. Go a little slower than you would in a big rush—this will prevent time-wasting mistakes. The clock is running from the time you enter the water until you cross the finish line at the end of the run; the seconds or even minutes spent changing your shoes, removing one set of clothing and putting on another all count just as much as the pace you set swimming, biking and running. Of course, NONE of it matters in the grand scheme of things, so try to remember that when you feel yourself getting a little uptight about all the rushing around going on. You're doing this for fun—never forget that. Let the immature, speedy youngsters get all stressed out and flummoxed—you can choose to be an island of serenity in a tempestuous sea of immaturity. Be a role model for everyone else.

It helps of course to arrive at the race site with plenty of time to set up, store what you will need and look around, sighting the familiar (and non-moveable landmarks, such as trees), noting where they are in relation to your bike location.

There are a wide range of other simple, logical steps to follow, nearly all of which the triathlon competitor will have mentally rehearsed prior to the event. If and when the unexpected occurs, as often is the case in triathlon as in life, the high performing triathlete will adapt and respond appropriately. Some of these odd possibilities can be anticipated (perhaps the strap on your helmet will seem difficult to snap into place); others are nearly unimaginable (you're lost in a sea of bikes!) but with a few deep breaths and an attitude of calm and reason, all can be managed with grace and panache.

Master the demands for an expeditious, enjoyable triathlon and you will add to your skills for managing change. While triathlon (and its sister sport of duathlon—a run/bike/run variation) is just a sport, a game and a pleasant, if demanding, diversion from the vital things in life (relationships, the quest for meaning and purpose and so on), it is a game that can help you discover many invaluable lessons applicable to the larger realm. You can apply these specific lessons to whatever you hold dear and consequential. Experiencing the sport and becoming skilled in managing transitions will help you with minor and major life changes. As with your performance in the two transition areas, you will come to face change with calm determination, wisdom, even humor at times, but always with style! You will appreciate the importance of planning for life changes, and your sense of control and personal efficacy will be greater than ever.

There are so many benefits to be gained from triathlon participation, and these opportunities account in part for its popularity. Join the movement. Consider becoming a triathlete, primarily because it is healthy and fun but also because it can be a sure way to learn how to deal effectively with change. Even if you choose to be one of those triathletes who does the sport strictly for fun, with no expectation of a medal, a plaque or a place on the national team, you can and will be a winner. You might enjoy a good triathlon book oriented to novices by physician/triathlete Steven Jonas. It is entitled *Triathloning for Ordinary Mortals* (Norton, NY, 2006.) and you will realize you don't have to finish first to win. Steve writes, "I can assure you that when you cross the finish line of your first race, regardless of your time, you will experience feelings of accomplishment and self-satisfaction unlike any you have experienced previously."

I hope you will act on this suggestion and give the sport a try. Visit the USAT website (www.usatriathlon.org). Play the game of triathlon, learn how to do a few graceful, stress-free and maybe even fast transitions and have yourself a winning life.

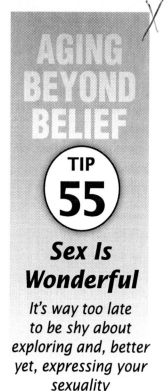

*I*s there one true way to deal with the oh-so-human drive to express your sexuality? No. Nor is there even a single wellness perspective on sexuality, or anything else. No one individual or organization should, in my view, try to set rules for everyone else on this delicious topic. We are too individualistic for that. The National Wellness Institute (NWI), the closest there is to a representative voice for wellness, does not issue position statements, proclamations or edicts on wellness, so I know they would not dare such a thing with respect to wellness and sexuality. I think it might be pretty cool if they did, provided their advice proved to be consistent with and reflective of my opinions. I fear, however, that they might stray, on occasions, from perspectives of which I approve. So, better the NWI keep out of this and leave it to me and everyone else, to decide for him/herself.

The drive for sex is a powerful human desire, perhaps the most powerful motive there is, next to the urge to plunder and pillage. (Kidding, though mankind has been known to do a great deal of both over time.) Napolean Hill, of *Think and Grow Rich* fame, believed sexual drive makes the imagination keener, the heart more courageous, the will more powerful, persistence greater and creative abilities more advanced. So strong and compelling is the desire for sexual contact that men freely risk reputation, liberty and even life itself to indulge their cravings for it. Nearly everyone, save a few of the holier than thou amongst us, like Pat Robertson and Jerry Falwell, for example, have a great interest in and energy for sex, whereas the drives for fitness, health, critical thinking and personal excellence seem much less powerful. Nothing changes as the years go by, except perhaps desire and performance. Come to think of it, that's pretty major, but that's no reason to not to make the best of what's left as long as it lasts.

I personally favor sexuality, and have been a supporter of this drive since the onset of puberty. I believe sexuality should be understood, discussed and embraced in an open manner, free of shame, guilt and moral restrictions. I think this is a wellness view, consistent with personal responsibility and the embrace of that which contributes to a high quality of life. I think religions have often made sex difficult if not dysfunctional, and that billions of people throughout history have had to endure ignorance about and suppression of their sexual nature. Among those who have been discouraged from indulging their sexual desires, even in responsible and considerate ways, are those considered "too old for that sort of thing." Balderdash.

Also, due to religious interpretations about sexual morality, governments have enforced all manner of restrictive rules and laws that constrain sexual expression for everyone.

An AUI wellness perspective on sexuality might well include the following elements:

1. A recognition that most people, especially seniors, have been subjected to much dysfunctional information during the formative years. For so many, the message about sex is "forget about it." It's too late. Most have internalized bizarre norms, customs, beliefs, traditions and practices hostile to sexuality of a wholesome, open and expressive nature. Thus, for many, the sad reality often is—it's too late. Hopefully, by adopting the idea that sex is inherently good and wholesome, and good for you, you can, over time, become less sexually suppressed and screwed up.

2. An orientation to getting your needs met to the extent possible without running afoul of your neighbors, co-workers or society in general. Do what you can to enjoy guilt-free sex without coming to the attention of the authorities.

3. A readiness to support grass roots initiatives for sexual

freedoms, including those that have no personal appeal. Examples might include strong support for gay and lesbian rights and opposition to restrictions on sexual expression, even if you personally don't wish to so express yourself. Examples include, but certainly are not limited to, such matters as pornography (still hard to define though most say they can recognize it), prostitution, strip joints, public nudity and so on).

4. The right of consenting adults to do as they like with their bodies. Unfortunately, if you live in Iran, Saudi Arabia, Alabama or other authoritarian theocracies or even a democratic society in which Republicans are a majority, forget it. Personally, I believe governments have no business in citizen's bedrooms. The role of the state should be the protection of the public good from physical injury. Morality is a private matter.

5. A devotion to healthy lifestyles, particularly regular daily exercise that keeps your sexuality at a high level of performance. Many studies have linked exercise to a better sex life. Besides the obvious fact that poor health does no favors for sexual functioning, exceptional fitness enhances performance and satisfaction in managing whatever contortions contribute to your pleasures. A Harvard School of Public Health study of 31,000 men showed the incidence of erectile dysfunction was 30 percent lower for men who were the most physically active. Another study at the University of British Columbia gave evidence of greater sexual response in women. Finally, if you exercise a lot and become terrifically fit, you will look more appealing to whomever you might want to have sex with.

Basically, sex is and should be seen as an enjoyable treat throughout life, a great way of meeting new people and a human right that gives life added meaning and purpose, at least while it's taking place.

Afterwards? Well, there's that lingering serenity for a spell, a sense of having accomplished something worthwhile and improved prospects for getting a good night's sleep.

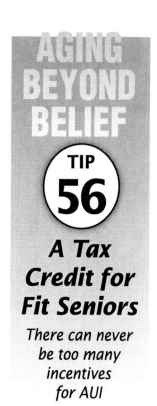

*I*f we seniors used our considerable influence with Congress to promote a modest tax credit for exercising personal responsibility rather than demanding more medical services, drugs and other handouts, we would do ourselves and all taxpayers a great service. This country has many serious problems to address, almost too numerous to mention, so I won't. Well, maybe a few, starting with the quality of our leaders, the absurdity of their policies, the obscene deficit being passed to future generations and the fact that most citizens are overweight, underfit, heavily medicated, superstitious and highly stressed. Other than that, things aren't so bad! Except for the so-called health care system, which, of course, is actually a fragmented, unsystematic and dysfunctional medical delivery hodgepodge.

All of which leads to my idea that the nation would benefit if Congress would pass a law granting a tax credit to seniors who have and continue to take good care of themselves. Here's why I think you might want to get behind this idea and use your considerable lobbying power as a member of AARP, a friend of a powerful politician, a big money donor or just some old codger or codgeress willing and able to make a fuss at public meetings.

We Americans pay $1.9 trillion for our medical system hodgepodge. We don't get good value for our money, though some privileged folks (members of Congress, federal employees) do enjoy generous medical benefit programs. Overall the results are not so good for most. While we pay more for medical care than citizens in other Western nations, we do not do better (e.g., live longer, get sick less often, have better infant mortality rates or other indices that reflect actual health status.) In addition, many (about 25 percent) Americans have little or no health insurance to help pay for medical expenses.

While it is not the entire solution, as everyone will eventually get sick and injured before dying of something, we could reduce medical costs dramatically if Americans were motivated and rewarded for staying well in the first place. Yes, genetics, environment and medical services matter, as does fate (sometimes a person is just in the wrong place at a bad time) but lifestyle is a category we can control. The influence of our behaviors on health status is vastly unappreciated and underemphasized by most policy makers (politicians).

Basically, the current situation can be summed up with the following axiom: Modern medicine is a wonderful thing, but there are two problems—we expect too much of it and too little of ourselves.

All of which is why I came up with the idea of tax credit subsidies for older Americans who take good care of themselves. By following a simple program of regular exercise, good diet and other disciplined practices known to optimize health and human performance, fit seniors boost their prospects to stay well in the first place. They do not unnecessarily burden the bloated medical system. They save Medicare a lot of money. They are good citizens, doing their part for America. Thus, it seems sensible for the government to provide attractive returns for such virtues. The benefits to society are substantial. That's why I think a nice tax subsidy is in order. Such an incentive would not only reward the virtuous seniors, but more importantly might motivate much of the rest of the population to follow their example. After all, they know that in time, they'll be old, too.

What do you think would happen if Congress passed laws that rewarded personal responsibility, daily exercise and good nutrition by seniors? I think the impact would be dramatic. Such incentives would lead to more behaviors that reduce the need for doctors, medications and health care professionals. It sure seems that way to me.

A wellness mindset that rewarded accountability would also discourage people from succumbing to temptations to blame someone else, make excuses, whine or wet their pants in the face of adversity. Let's promote policies that offer alternatives to the sorry status quo, to complacency, to mediocrity and to self-pity, boredom and slothfulness.

Besides exercise and fitness, nutrition and stress management, a national campaign with suitable tax and other incentives could encourage other wellness qualities. Among them might be critical thinking, a conscious quest for added meaning and purpose in daily life, the development of greater emotional intelligence and more tolerance, humor, play and effective relationships.

Let's have a changed focus, not on more medical care or more drugs or more cures but more guidance and support for appreciating what it means to be a healthy senior, as opposed to just not being sick.

Let's have a country that celebrates and rewards those who do just that. To recall the wise words of an aging Arthur Godfrey, "I'm proud to be paying taxes. The only thing is—I could be just as proud for half the money."

*T*his is particularly applicable when such communications are by e-mail. We're all inundated with urban legends (UL's). Amazingly, many otherwise sensible people assume these tales to be factual—and pass them along. Often, the tales are alleged to have happened to "a friend of a friend." Documentation of the information is either missing or inaccurate. How come the friends of someone's friend seem to have lives that are so much more interesting, if not bizarre, than the friends themselves?

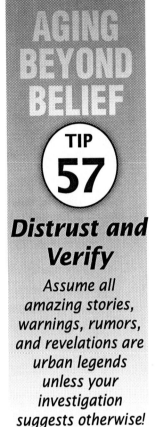

TIP

57

Distrust and Verify

Assume all amazing stories, warnings, rumors, and revelations are urban legends unless your investigation suggests otherwise!

UL's are a lot like movies "BASED on actual events!" What does "based on actual events" really mean? Isn't everything, in one way or another, based somehow on something sort of similar, in a way? When the credit line in a movie makes this claim, you can be sure that the plot is unrecognizable from the original event, grossly distorted, wildly exaggerated and ridiculously sensationalized. The movie "King Kong" is based on an actual event, I suppose. Apes are actually taken from jungles to be put on display by humans. So, "King Kong" is based on actual events. Sure, and the check is probably in the mail.

To help slow the spread of UL's, at least among those on your mailing list, here are a few tips for smoking out UL's before they waste your time and add to the continued dumbing-down of America.

UL's are with us because so many people are undereducated, poor thinkers, superstitious, brain-dead and plain foolish. Also, they flourish because so many WANT certain legends to be accepted, especially if they support a moral lesson or a political view favored by the person spamming everyone with it. Also, many people are too lazy to check the status of UL's at Snopes.com or other sites devoted to UL assessment. There are so many other explanations—here are a few more:

- Some tales are fun, amusing or even amazing— "What the heck—let's see how my retired buddies react to this," could be a motive for sending some legends around.

- A lot of conspiracy kooks use UL's to boost their worldview, as do religious proselytizers to show that Jesus really does hate gays, that the Rapture is coming or that George Bush was nominated and elected by God.

- Occasionally, a UL turns out to be true, or at least grounded in fact (though embellished), such as the one at Snopes about "My Retirement Plan." (This story was last updated on March 15, 2005. It describes how "some people have eschewed retirement homes in favor of living on cruise ships." The full story is at www.snopes.com/travel/trap/retire.asp.

At Snopes and other UL assessment sites, a cute signaling device, like red ("Stop") and green ("Go") colors, are posted to distinguish the bogus to the mostly true suspected UL's. In any event, there are several things to look for if a message comes into your inbox that looks like a UL.

- Consider the source. Do you know who sent it? Is he or she a sensible person, or a lunatic? If the sender does not have impeccable credentials, be suspicious. If he/she does, be suspicious anyway.

- Use a reliable website for checking out tales that interest you enough to investigate. (Most ULs deserve an immediate deletion.) I suggest the urban legends website at About. com, but Snopes http://www.snopes.com/ and others are also excellent.

- Does the tale begin with a suspicious assurance that "this is a true story?" That is a good sign it's not! Ditto if the sender, anonymous, insists that "this really happened to a friend of a friend or the wife of a co-worker or my brother's housekeeper's son," etc.

- If it ends with a warning that your teeth will fall out or you will go straight to hell if you don't send it to everyone in your address book in one minute, or otherwise hints that awful things have happened to those who did NOT forward the rumor, hit the delete button immediately. It was, no doubt about it, sent by a crazy person.

- If the story sounds familiar or has come from a lot of different sources but with varying details and circumstances or other "facts," it's a stinker, for sure. While you can't believe everything you read in the newspapers, the fact that a story has not been reported in any of them is not a good sign, either.

- Respect your own baloney detector. You can sense if the evidence to support a story smells like a dead fish long out of water. If there are "commonsense reasons to disbelieve it," activate this common sense.

- The best of all guides, I suspect, is the one you have surely heard many times and which can be ignored only at great peril: If a story seems too good, too horrible, too improbable or too funny to be true, well, come on now, you know it isn't!

Rene Descartes declared "All is to be doubted" (De omnibus dubitandum) and Dilbert (Scott Adams) asked, "When did ignorance become a point of view?" What's more, be aware that "A witty saying (or tale) proves nothing" (Voltaire) and that "The beginning of wisdom is found in doubting; by doubting we come to the question, and by seeking we may come upon the truth." (Pierre Abelard) One more thing, while I'm on this theme—"Always look on the bright side of life." (Monty Python)

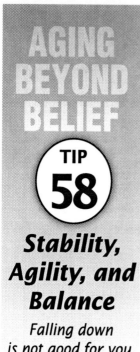

AGING BEYOND BELIEF

TIP 58

Stability, Agility, and Balance

Falling down is not good for you, so take steps to prevent it

*F*alls are usually no big deal during the early and even middle years of life. Some are, of course, but most of us, especially guys, grow up playing sports where falling is part of the game, as is the process of actually inducing falls among each other (like when playing football). But, falling down for senior adults, particularly those with limited mobility to begin with, is a serious matter. Doing so may lead to broken bones, which will interfere with your active wellness lifestyle and put a crimp in your social life. Consider these precautions:

• Create a safe home environment that reduces the risks of falls.

• Install devices that make life easier, if and when needed, such as grab bars and railings in strategic locations.

• Make sure your home and work environments are well lighted.

• Have your vision and hearing checked regularly.

• Keep plenty of Viagra or other safe, performance enhancing aids on hand, just in case. (No, this tip has nothing to do with preventing falls.)

In the first sentence of this tip, above, I used the phrase "senior adult." What, exactly, is a senior adult? When does the word "senior" officially attach to the word "adult" in references to you? There is no official word on this or consensus, but here are indicators of when you have gone over to "the other side," so to speak.

• When you wife says, "Let's go upstairs and make love, you reply: Honey, I can't do both!"

• When your friends compliment you on your new alligator shoes—and you're barefoot.

- When the porn you bring home is called "Debby Does Dialysis."

- When your doctor doesn't give you x-rays anymore, but just holds you up to the light.

- When a babe catches your fancy and your pacemaker sets off the garage door.

- When you remember the time the Dead Sea was only sick.

(These lines have been attributed to varied comedians, largely because they stole them from each other.)

Naturally, falling down is no laughing matter; serious efforts should be made to prevent such disasters. Outside areas can be designed to be safer, as well, though this requires public action beyond the initiative of individual seniors. Examples of safe designs are smooth and attractive walking paths that separate cyclists, skaters and rollerbladers. Of course, some senior adults ARE bikers, skaters, and rollerbladers, but such senior adults are vigorous and less needful of protection.

The number one safeguard against falls is to create, sustain, and continuously fine-tune a healthy lifestyle. This will enable you to enter senior adulthood in top form and to extend the period of quality life to the greatest extent possible.

However, even if you are the wellest person on earth or a serious candidate for such an award, if ever one should be created, the fact is you are still going to grow old, eventually—assuming you don't get hit by a bus or carry genes programmed to do you in before you reach a state of semi-frailty, senility, or worse. And no matter how much you exercise to build bone and cardiovascular strength, remain flexible, work out vigorously on a daily basis to insure muscular support for bones, and otherwise do all that self-management skill building and behavior invites, at some point these suggestions will prove beneficial.

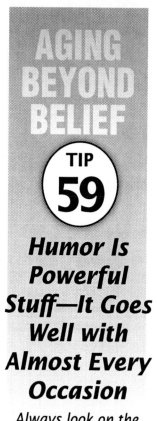

Humor Is Powerful Stuff—It Goes Well with Almost Every Occasion

Always look on the light side of life

*S*cholars have said as much for centuries. Humor can be artfully applied to nearly all situations. If you doubt this, consider something as profoundly unfunny as the Holocaust! A scholarly paper ("Humor in the Holocaust: Its Critical, Cohesive, and Coping Functions") by John Morreall provides specific instances of humor's comforting grace even during times of unimaginable horror. Morreall suggests that Western culture generally shies from tempering tragedy with humor in favor of restricting mirth to matters light in nature. Morreall reminds us that, "the ancient Greeks, Shakespeare, and other dramatists took their comedy more seriously. They realized that comedy is not a 'time out' from the real world; rather it provides another perspective on that world." Just so, it seems to me. Conrad Hyers said comedy expresses "a stubborn refusal to give tragedy ... the final say." In fact, humor is akin to religion in the sense that it is a diversionary tactic helping mankind deal with tragedy and evil—and thereby ward off despair, for a little while. Once rational faculties set in again, despair returns as the only logical choice—until more humor (or piety) can be invented.

For Shakespeare, unlike the politically correct of our time, no subject was off-limits, not even the gods. I should say, particularly not the gods. What's more, Mark Twain demonstrated that comedy was too important to be confined to the frivolous. It was Twain who wrote, "The secret source of humor itself is not joy but sorrow." (*The Mysterious Stranger*)

Humor relies on surprise, juxtaposition and incongruity. A humorous thread goes along one track and suddenly, at the punch line, ends in another. Our train of thought leaves the track and, if the jolt is enjoyable, a laugh or smile ensues. Morreall shows that "Holocaust humor" served three main functions:

1. The critical function: It focused attention on what was wrong and sparked resistance to it.

2. The cohesive function: It created solidarity in those laughing together at the oppressors.

3. The coping function: It helped the oppressed get through their suffering without going insane.

So, next time you start to feel sorry for yourself or otherwise get a little bummed or stressed, seek refuge with a natural chemical fix (in other words, a seratonin brain surge) by finding a way to humor yourself. If Viktor Frankl and other residents of Holocaust concentration camps could do it, you should be able to manage the feat. David Nathan, author of *The Laughtermakers*, viewed laughter as part of the human survival kit.

A condition somewhat less dramatic but more universal than the Holocaust, for which humor provides a momentary escape valve of sorts, is aging. This "condition" humor can't cure but a good sense of humor does offer many effective short-term treatments. Humor is a lot less expensive and/or invasive than some of the other "cures," such as face lifts, breast implants, flashy sports cars, younger lovers, training for and participating in triathlons and hormone injections.

For a delightful overview on the dynamics and social consequences of satirical humor, visit Richard Dawkins website. Look around, then click on the January 7, 2007 link to Channel 4's production about the making of the Monty Python movie, "The Life of Brian." The video has clips of the movie and interviews with persons involved in the controversies surrounding the movie before and after its release. There is much to be learned in all this about the role of humor relative to freedom of speech.

At the end of the documentary, Terry Gilliam observes, "Comedy is not particularly difficult. You can get laughs doing any number of things, but to get laughs at an intelligent level about an important subject, oooh, that's good."

I'm guessing you would agree.

*W*hether hard-earned or easy come thanks to good fortune and your unmitigated brilliance, you have a right to be tight with your money. Aristotle advised, "To give away money is an easy matter and in any man's power. But to decide to whom to give it, and how large, and when, and for what purpose and how, is neither in every man's power nor an easy matter."

If a friend, relative or business associate asks you to donate to what he/she believes is a good cause, do you always feel obligated to do so? Are you often too uncomfortable about the situation to say, "No?"

Consider making a choice next time you are in this situation. The choice is this: "Do I want to feel uncomfortable, pressured and more or less obligated to contribute, or not?" That's step one. Make "not" your choice.

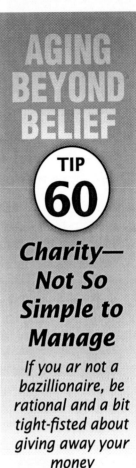

TIP

60

Charity— Not So Simple to Manage

If you ar not a bazillionaire, be rational and a bit tight-fisted about giving away your money

You have a right not to allow others to make you uncomfortable. Exercise your right to decide what cause, charity or campaign, if any, you support. It's really OK to decline to give to a cause embraced by someone else, even a person who is important to you. If it strains the relationship a bit, well, the tension is a fair price for wisely managing whatever resources you have available, if any, to simply give away.

I came to this conclusion the other day when a friend tried to hit me up for a donation. By E-mail, he announced that his wife was running a marathon for a disease and wanted me (and others who know him or her) to pay his wife to do so (via a donation to HER cause, not necessarily mine). As with so many running and multi-sport events, the wife would be gathering pledges for miles run to be given to professional fund-raisers hired to assist the disease-fighting non-profit agency that would eventually receive what was left of the donated funds.

I could have ignored it, that is, kept my mouth/keyboard still and just let it go away. But nooooooooooo, I had to shoot off a reaction to this. This was my message:

Most people asked to donate money because a friend is doing some event in honor of a cause—and raising money at the same time, either just do it for the friend or ignore the request. I don't want to do either. I prefer to explain why not because if the situation were reversed, I'd prefer a forthright response to being ignored after making a personal request.

We know many people doing X or Y race for causes A through Z. It would get expensive to give to the event/cause of all who ask, and an energy drain even to ponder who to or who not to support. I surely could not support them all—there are too many. Besides, my wife and I do a lot of races—the idea of paying into the charities of others to honor THEIR races seems a stretch. I think the idea of paying for someone else to collect money for a cause by running miles and such appeals most to non-athletes who view doing a marathon or triathlon as a big deal. Such feats are sensible things, but not a sound basis for allocating a portion of fixed/limited charitable dollars amongst a very large list of individuals and organizations, all doing fund raising on behalf of many worthy causes. Besides, the charities that put these fund raisers together are often themselves big business operations, and I suspect that they draw off a good portion of the funds raised to support, what else, more fund raising promotions—and the salaries and expenses that make all the requisite organizing and fund-raising possible.

Maybe it's better if people just donate to the causes they want to support.

What do you think? Does this make sense? Maybe I'm just cheap. Basically, I prefer a more rational approach to giving and recommend the same to you. A nice note of explanation is good but should not be mandatory.

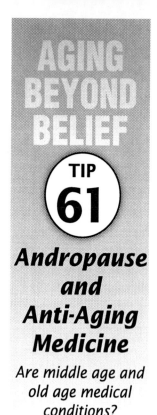

AGING BEYOND BELIEF

TIP

61

*Andropause
and
Anti-Aging
Medicine*

*Are middle age and
old age medical
conditions?*

*A*re testosterone injections, surgeries and other "treatments" for symptoms of aging miracle-like advances in science, or medical hucksterism more hazardous than hopeful?

I'm often asked, "Is it fair to equate middle age with ignorance and apathy." My answer never varies: "I don't know and I don't care." Well, the complexities of the issue at hand are daunting. Old age is for real, but middle age is illusory. Of course, whether this statement is true or false, profound or absurd depends—on the meaning of terms. What IS old age? What about middle age? What IS Andropause and what, exactly, is anti-aging medicine and what does the evidence show, so far? As you have surely heard more than once, the reality for most is, "I can't define it but I know it when I see it or, in this case, when I feel it."

Curiously, there are some pretty good informal definitions of middle and old ages. An elderly lady once told me that middle age is "when your husband tells you he is having an affair, and you want to know if it's going to be catered." Someone else said, "Middle age is when you remove the mirror over your bed—and replace it with a poster of the food pyramid. (I removed my ceiling mirror recently. There was something about that message on the side that made guests nervous—you know the one: "Objects in mirror are closer than they appear.")

All this is intended as good fun. If we can't change something, well, why not just laugh about it, or at least try to smirk at life's slings and arrows when we can? However, when a new medical specialty evolves to deal with aging in the middle and later years, an approach at odds with established scientific medicine involving immense financial, health and life quality implications, then it's time to get somewhat serious. At such times, we are wise to try our best to understand what can and what cannot be done to influence the aging process with this new strategy, if anything. Meet "Andropause" or "male menopause," a complex of conditions associated with the gradual decline in sexuality, mood overall energy, skin elasticity, organ size and other, unpleasant changes associated with aging.

Andropause encompasses a variety of medical prevention and treatment strategies. An entire industry has grown in the past decade or so to address concerns identified under the Andropause banner.

Now the key question for all interested in AUI of wellness lifestyles becomes: Is this a legitimate field, with evidence-based protocols, or not? Should you work with "anti-aging" doctors to prevent and/or treat Andropause-related problems?

How do I know? I'm not a doctor—I just play one when writing books.

No, seriously, it's too early to be sure. There is a lot of anecdotal information about older folks who have benefited from anti-aging strategies. However, this is as reliable as paid advertising, though it's quite different. There are and always have been lots of sincere and dramatic testimonials about miracles, too, but this is faith-based information, not solid evidence grounded in objective scientific analysis. Andropause remedies and approaches have not been shown to be beneficial in controlled, independent trials with results published in peer-reviewed journals.

So, I'm not saying there is no value in the Andropause movement but a lot of hype attends the subject. Personally, I hope it will prove to be the best thing to come along since aspirin, or better yet, wellness lifestyles. However, I prefer to wait for more evidence before signing up for testosterone injections or other Andropause treatments. I think you should wait, also, while informing yourself about the issues. Be prepared to do a lot of reading and other searching—this is a huge area that will get bigger in time, for better or worse.

Personally, at this point, I'm a skeptic. Is a lower testosterone level a unique condition, or just another symptom of getting older, like hair loss, wrinkled skin and the urge to take ocean cruises? I'm leaning against the whole idea of Andropause, despite the anecdotes from Sandy and others I highly regard. I think "cures," such as facelifts, flashy sports cars, breast implants and hormone injections for battling aging are ultimately futile. (Of course, everything is ULTIMATELY futile, including efforts to breathe.) However, I admit I'm not entirely consistent about this sort of thing. I always appreciate breast implants and what's there not to like about flashy sports cars?

I do have a few questions about Andropause treatments. Do anti-aging doctors also emphasize healthy lifestyles to patients? Are patients urged to exercise vigorously consistent with their capabilities, to eat well, manage stress and undertake other health-enhancing initiatives? I suspect some of the attention to Andropause is related to the aging of baby boomers. Not unlike generations who aged before them, baby boomers don't like the signs of growing old—but unlike their predecessors, they demand something be done about it. "How could life do this to me, after all I have done for life itself?" This seems to be the lament of the Andro generation. There is no medication that does not have side effects. Statins have the potential to wreck the liver. Like many other "miracle" drugs, they have been around too short a time for all the information to be definitive - and they bring in WAY too much money for the drug companies for them to be terribly anxious to find out.

Books, lectures, websites and anything else focused on a disease, illness or condition of dis-ease (as in Andropause) always draw more attention than similar products and services for wellness. That's just the way it is. That's also why doctors make the big bucks. There is a lot more interest in sickness and discomfort (e.g., incontinence) than wellness. People seem willing to do heaps more to deal with a discomfort than to experience a pleasure. Self-managed, self-disciplined individuals do not search websites looking for confirmation from wellness gurus that they're doing the right thing. Most surfers are looking for solutions or something miraculous to take away their pain. Or, they seek commiseration for the fact that they're getting older. Not you, of course.

Again, I acknowledge that I could be full of evil smelling stuffing in not embracing this emerging field for extending life quality. My friend Sandy Scott, whom you encountered in previous tips (see # 34), is an enthusiast for the reality of Andropause and particularly for the benefits he personally experienced from taking anti-aging medical interventions. He told me many stories, including one about a 70-year-old female friend who underwent a tummy tuck and a complete facelift. He said she looks and feels like a million dollars and, more important, that the surgery vastly enhances her mental outlook and quality of life. He added, "You can do sit-ups until you melt, but if you are genetically programmed to have a spare tire, you simply ain't getting rid of it in any way that I know, except surgery. Another friend, an accomplished masters swimmer who spent lots of time in his Speedo, had been quite self-conscious about the one part of his body that was not fit looking—his midsection. Liposuction saved the day, and he tells the story to anyone that will listen because it has so enhanced his life (as he sees it)."

Sandy's personal experience and extensive research on treatment protocols have led him to support anti-aging hormone and other medical strategies. He claims such approaches counter the adverse effects of aging for many, including depression and bone and muscle loss. In his view, simple testosterone (gel) treatments sometimes change lives. While acknowledging that long-term studies have not been done, he said, "I would rather roll the dice than be depressed every other day." He even defended pharmaceutical companies, saying, "In many instances they ARE bad guys, but they also do incredible things to enhance healthy lifestyles. I, for example, could never get my total cholesterol below a bit over 200 through serious dieting and intense exercise. The miracle of statins have given me one of the best blood lipid profiles you have ever seen with no negative side effects."

Well, there you have it—another instance wherein the best course is to study the issues, get lots of opinions, weigh the evidence and make an informed choice. As Sandy concluded, "a very complicated, controversial, endless subject." But, just as Robert Frost had his promises to keep, I have my tips to finish before I sleep, so I WILL end the subject here. I'll also pass the responsibility for deciding, in your case, where it belongs. To you.

You will have to struggle, at times, as everyone must. Whether you eventually prosper will depend on your own actions and resources. Don't waste time dwelling upon condolences, however well-intended. Focus instead on what you can do to overcome adversity, and move forward. The quality of your life is in your hands. It is up to you.

I suggest you view adversity as part of life, as something that happens to everyone, even you! Defined as "a condition of suffering, affliction or a calamitous or disastrous experience," we all come face-to-face with it throughout life, and more often than before as the years pile up. No doubt, you are quite familiar with adversity; you might have wondered, now and then, how come you are "visited" by the experience so often!

Adversity and Resilience

Resolve to regroup and return, stronger than ever

The AUI of a wellness lifestyle perspective on adversity is that reestablishing interest, vitality and excitement in life is your responsibility, in good times and bad. Into every life a little and, occasionally, a lot of rain (adversity) will fall. In the long haul, and the short run as well, it will be your attitude toward adversity more than the calamity itself that will affect how successful you are in coping, managing and then moving along in life toward better times. A wellness way of seeing things will improve the chances that you will move ahead, sooner rather than later, stronger than you were before.

There are little adversities and great calamities. The principles for coping, adapting and managing that I just summarized apply equally in all cases. However, it is a lot easier to deal with the little adversities than the grand catastrophes. To give a personal example regarding adversities in the first category, I might mention the frustrations of most if not all senior athletes, namely, injuries and performance disappointments. Though there is little at stake, except ego and a preference to have fun in certain ways, it is so tempting to feel sorry for myself, to wallow in self-pity and to look for someone else to blame! Doing so is dysfunctional, since it does not entail accepting the reality that you must adapt and choose constructive action. Accepting the inevitability of adversity and assuming accountability for doing something makes the challenging event or circumstance itself less troublesome.

During adversity, you will be tested by nature, the gods, fate or whatever. Personally, I think you are better off if you choose not to think that it is God or the Devil doing the testing. Surely if either or both exist, they have more important things to do than to mess around with your life! Don't take such things personally. It's part of life.

Remember, JFK was right—life IS unfair—always has been, always will be. Get used to it. Think of your senior years as filled with tests, daily. Part of the testing process is adapting to these challenges without a diminution in the quality of your life. These tests are basically pass or fail. You pass by figuring out ways to remain as healthy as is possible, to continue finding some measure of joy in living, staying engaged, and finding reasons for getting enthused now and then. While you cannot know the nature of future challenges in the form of adversities, you can mitigate them a bit by knowing they are as certain as sunrises and sunsets. Accept this reality and better position yourself to deal with life as it is and to do your best to look on the bright side of life.

If it were easy, everyone would be doing it. With a wellness perspective, it will be easier to regain the momentum needed to get back to your sense for adventure and quest for the best life you can fashion under difficult circumstances.

*T*wo wellness promoters believe "icantdoit" is the reality for most people and urge seekers of healthier lifestyles, young and old, to adopt an "icantdoit" point of view—at least for a while. I'm one of them; the other is Grant Donovan, an Australian colleague.

The Reality of "Icantdoit"

It won't be easy, but do it anyway

Grant and I came to this position reluctantly, and we did so over a long period of time, agonizing about it and gnashing our teeth (figuratively speaking). After all, like other wellness promoters, we were cheerleaders for healthy lifestyles. We much preferred the standard, "you can do whatever you set your mind to doing," style of advice. Unfortunately, our research and experience eventually convinced us that this is simply not true. People can't succeed at all, unless they are exceptional, heroic or aware of and prepared for the difficulties of sustaining good intentions. If it were easy to live well, people would do it. They would succeed at health promotion. Clearly, they don't, which you might have noticed if you look around (e.g., 64 percent of Americans are overweight or even obese).

So, we decided we could be more effective if we urged folks to "stop tilting at windmills." Don Quixote tilted at windmills, and where did it get him? We decided not to fool around about this "icantdoit" reality. We wrote and otherwise communicated messages like, Why bust your buns trying to do that which is beyond your reach? Accept your mediocrity. Deal with the obvious and remind yourself of how things really are. Repeat after me: "I can't do it." And, of course, we explained why this is so in great detail.

We made the case that, if you COULD put into practice and sustain healthy choices, you would have done so long ago. You would have accepted more responsibility for the quality of your life. You would have exercised vigorously on a regular basis, eaten well, managed

189

stress, practiced critical thinking and done the innumerable things you knew were in your best interests. However, insurmountable barriers stood in the way. Dr. Donovan and I listed over thirty such barriers, which included genetics, environment, insufficient education, lack of persistence, ill health, irrationality, lack of cooperation, insufficient ambition, poor self discipline, negative personality and so on. We reviewed the literature that supported these findings, including the work of Napoleon Hill, author of the 1937 classic *Think and Grow Rich*. You can read at least twenty essays on the nature of our "icantdoit" philosophy at www.seekwellness. com/wellness/icantdoit.htm

In any event, these are some of the reasons we have been telling people to respect the reality of "icantdoit." It may seem that we are discouraging folks from pursuing wellness and a better life, but that is not the case. Not at all. On the contrary, we simply decided that an adherence to common decencies mandated that we tell the truth, as we (reluctantly) came to view the reality of achieving a wellness lifestyle worthy of the concept. However, "icantdoit" is a beginning, not the end, of a preferred strategy. It is an insight intended to guide living well and, in the present case, aging under the influence of a wellness lifestyle. It is not a concession, nor is it an acceptance of defeat. Just the opposite—it is an essential first step to success. That is the purpose of our "icantdoit" message. It is an introduction. The best part is step two.

Step two involves setting modest objectives, after fully appreciating the difficulties and taking account of inventive ways to overcome the many barriers to sustaining wellness lifestyles. These steps might involve a planning process, a basic awareness of the research relating to your goals, the creation and nurturing of cultural supports, the shaping of environments that facilitate changes you seek and all manner of additional strategies that take account of success factors described by Napoleon Hill and others.

Accept the notion "I can't do it" and, counter intuitively, it becomes easier to get on with your life. Then you can do what is possible and be grateful and appreciative of every advance. If you do "it"—regardless of what "it" might be, AFTER accepting "icantdoit" at both intellectual and emotional levels, the outcome will surely provide a satisfying treat. Thereafter, you will realize other advances that once fell in the "I can't do it category." Keep the bar low and don't try too much. Without the baggage of fear of failure or similar anxieties, great and small, that burden the quest for ambitious goals, you'll IMPROVE your prospects to do it. Whatever the "it" is that you decide upon.

When you show those who want you to say, "Icantdoit," that you can do it, nobody will be happier about it than Grant Donovan and yours truly. Good luck. Go for it—all the way.

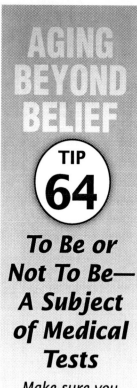

To Be or Not To Be— A Subject of Medical Tests

Make sure you clearly need a given test or screening

*E*arlier this year, I had an MRI. The objective—to diagnose knee pain (meniscus tear was suspected) and enable an informed course of action (arthroscopy). Given the costs and risks of most medical procedures, I did a lot of independent study on the need for this procedure. In short order, I decided that, if I wanted to run again, it was almost certainly a good bet and a worthy investment. Few critics of the medical system concerned with waste, fraud, redundancy and other abuses oppose all testing. But how might consumers distinguish necessary, prudent testing from the rest? Is there really a problem with too much testing, too many unnecessary procedures?

Maybe, depending on whom you believe. A few years ago, doctors at a for-profit hospital in California performed unnecessary tests AND unnecessary operations on healthy people ("How One Hospital Benefited on Questionable Operations," *New York Times*, August 12, 2003.) The Redding institution and two of its top doctors carried out "tens of thousands of diagnostic tests (and) thousands of surgical coronary procedures." The hospital's owner, Tenet Healthcare, agreed to pay $54 million for unnecessary heart procedures and operations on hundreds of healthy patients; for years, lawsuits and criminal investigations continued.

Amazing? Yes, but not so surprising considering the incentives in place that encourage testing and medical procedures. "If in doubt, cut it out—and go to the bank to deposit more money earned," is the norm in our dysfunctional medical system, some advise. Such alarmists urge caution and objective third party assessments to protect against falling prey to abuses.

Uwe Reinhardt, a health care economist, remarked (in the above noted Times piece): "I sometimes just shake my head at the American system, where the financial intent is almost cleverly designed to create mischief. For administrators, it creates a conflict of interest when they're trying to deliver the numbers at the same time that doctors are saying the hospital is doing too much cardiac surgery." One built-in problem that encourages reckless testing and unnecessary procedures (but generates revenues for hospitals and promotions and rewards for doctors) is the system itself. Reinhardt notes, "financial markets, which drive Tenet and other investors in the system, reward double-digit earnings growth from hospital companies." Such growth is hard to sustain under normal conditions (in other words, conservative medical practices.) Reinhardt: "The hospital industry is by its very nature a mature industry. It is not a high-margin business. It can't be a growth industry like some Internet company. That is just unreasonable."

One of the "best performers" or rainmakers at the Redding hospital conducted over 35,000 catheterizations, a sum other cardiologists found remarkable. Curiously, the doctor accused of excessive testing and operations told associates his decision to become a doctor "had been dictated to him by God when he was a boy." However, the Times article did not reveal whether the good doctor believed God dictated all those catheterizations.

The doctors who performed tests and operations were paid handsomely and treated well by the hospital administration, with helicopter rides to golf courses and other perks affirming their power and prestige. For doctors bringing in the big bucks, "normal checks and balances did not seem to apply." Federal investigators later discovered that the highest performing doctor was not board certified in cardiology or internal medicine, yet headed the Cardiology Care Committee. This peer review group responsible for program quality rarely met.

After numerous reports of recommended bypass surgeries that were found unwarranted in second and third opinions and a spate of lawsuits, the FBI raided the hospital. Accusations of unnecessary surgery and gaming the Medicare system were leveled and the Department of Health and Human Services audited all Tenet hospitals. Tenet's top executives, and those at the Redding hospital, are gone. Medicare payments at the hospital fell $23 million the first quarter of the year of the investigations.

What are the lessons here? I can think of five, for starters. All promote a cautious relationship with the medical system:

1. Consider the risks of medical testing. A worst-case is you could be given an incorrect diagnosis, and channeled into an operating room unnecessarily.

2. Question the need for tests and be reluctant to submit to them. While the common reaction to being told "everything is fine" after undergoing medical testing is usually, "Wow—that's great news," the fact is that "everything is fine" means you just wasted your time and money and put up with pain and discomfort to gain peace of mind! You want "peace of mind?" There are often safer, cheaper and more sensible ways to secure it.

3. Your own checking. Maybe the risks of testing are worth the aggravations for assurance that you don't have something awful. If tests reveal a problem, then they were not a waste of money or the hours that could have been spent doing other, more pleasant things. Some tests are certainly of value and nothing herein should dissuade you from having them done. Invest the energy needed for good choices.

4. Recognize that some preventive screenings and tests do make sense. One to consider is a colonoscopy, which independent medical experts advise every 3 to 5 years for everyone over 50. Colon cancers develop from non-cancerous polyps, which can be removed during the procedure. If a cancer is detected and removed before spreading, chances of survival are

good, whereas the prognosis is usually not good by the time symptoms appear. Colon cancer is the third most common cancer death among both men and women. Of course, a wellness lifestyle reduces the risk of colon cancer, particularly the practice of enjoying five to nine servings daily of vegetables along with the discipline of regular exercise.

5. Contribute as you can, in your own fashion, to modest reforms. What you do will, in the aggregate, make a difference, however modest. Of course, if you have any political influence, you can make a greater difference by supporting reforms in national health care incentives. Reforms might begin with a focus on the big picture—looking at a massive shift from the provision of medical care to the promotion of healthy lifestyles. The Redding doctors and administrators were only working the system, which invited testing and invasive procedures.

In summary, beware—do NOT trust. Verify! In addition, look after yourself by practicing a wellness lifestyle.

TIP

65

Doubt Is a Virtue

In this and other mostly free countries, you have a right to doubt—exercise it

*I*f you were a citizen of Iran, Saudi Arabia, or any other theocracy and/or dictatorship, you could not doubt our leaders, at least not publicly—AND remain free. For many of us in this country and throughout the West, the right to doubt is seen as crucial to our freedom. I believe it is also vital to our prospects for sustaining a wellness lifestyle.

How important do you regard freedom to doubt and otherwise to think and act critically in a public way? What if you found it difficult or dangerous to express doubt in the context of prevailing sentiments to go along and conform? Would that be a major concern for you? Is it a big deal—or only a theoretical issue, as you see it?

I recommend you view this right to question authority and to challenge claims of expertise as a right worth protecting. It's important that you do so, for certain things are happening in America that require a vigilance on the part of the public to protect this right to doubt, to question and to dissent.

The need is something caused in part by the irresponsibility of the mass media in exploiting the public taste for nonsense, the ineffectiveness of public education and the irrationality of the American world-view oriented to supernatural thinking. In summary, Americans are taught WHAT, not HOW to think. To be effective at expressing doubt on any topic, consider this mini-code of personal behavior:

1. Be nice to everybody.

2. Say whatever you think.

3. Take nothing personally—and try not to take your own opinions too seriously.

4. Consider that religion is too consequential to leave in the proverbial closet—express your doubts about it, if you have any—and do the same with respect to sex and politics.

5. Remind yourself that tolerance and civility do not require everyone to agree with or pretend to have no opinion about matters you find ridiculous or jejune.

6. Let others know that you are not out to convince them to think the way you think. Adopt an attitude that doubt is just a process by which you entertain yourself, and that you don't give a hoot if others believe what you believe. People are easier to take when it's clear they don't want to convert, save or reform.

7. Be sure to display a similar attitude toward others. Among other benefits, it's an effective stress avoider.

I can't be sure of it but, based on their writings and what others have written about them, I'm ready to bet (a small sum) that all the following characters would like this tip: Confucius, Socrates, Plato, Augustine, Epicurus and Diogenes, Maimonides, Job and Ecclesiastes, Newton, Descartes, Pascal, Galileo, Spinoza, Robespierre, Paine, Jefferson, JS Mill, Harriet Taylor, Frederick Douglas, Susan B. Anthony, Lucretius, Ovid, Keats, Dickenson, Marx, Freud, Nietzsche, Edison, Sanger and Twain. These people were all heteroclites! A heteroclite is someone who deviates from the ordinary rule; an eccentric—one who is unconventional; a maverick. It's never too late in life to cultivate good qualities, and challenging "certainties" surely is one of them. Mark C. Taylor, a religion and humanities professor at Williams College and author of "Mystic Bones," in an op-ed piece for the *New York Times* entitled, "The Devoted Student," December 21, 2006, suggested "the task of thinking and teaching, especially in an age of emergent fundamentalisms, is to cultivate a faith in doubt that calls into question every certainty."

The next time some politician goes on about the "sanctity" of marriage, "God bless America," pray for this or pray for that or anything else that triggers your doubt reflex, think about how fortunate we (still) are that we can beg to differ, give voice to dissent, think critically (aloud) and take exception to traditional, majority opinion. We can, if we find it necessary for our own approaches to wellness, exercise our freedom to take issue with anything we believe is at odds with reason, evidence, experience, common sense or just our bare-nekked opinion, rational or otherwise.

*N*ext time someone asks, "How are you doing?"—say, "Wonderful, could not be better," or something like that, no matter how you're doing. The reason? Optimism, that is, looking on the bright side, could help you live longer—according to researchers who studied this phenomenon over a period of 30 years.

Naturally, this will have little or more likely no effect if you are at the end of the rope, or otherwise in a terminal situation. Being or pretending to be optimistic does NOT cure heart disease, reverse trauma, eliminate cancer or anything of that nature. Trying to be optimistic, cheerful or other than depressed is still sensible and good, if challenging. And it can affect your mood and feeling states. All this is self-evident, but worth mentioning. You never know—somebody might erroneously assume I'm suggesting that optimism cures disease or prevents death—or something else rather bizarre along such lines.

Before I tell you about the study, let me go back a bit to the 70s, when I began promoting wellness lifestyles.

I was in California at the time. I heard lots of hippy-dippy, holistic types go on about how great this was and that was and so on—all positive talk, even if discussing a hurricane or earthquake. It did not matter among the hippy-dippys—they gave everything a positive spin. They acted as if professing a belief would make it so. Most, in fact, took the idea of looking on the bright side to extremes. Repeat enough affirmations and you can have abundance, love, a baby or whatever you want, reason notwithstanding.

Well, maybe I was too cynical. Now research comes along suggesting the bright side people may have been on to something. An Ohio longitudinal study concerning aging and retirement, which started in

A Positive Spin

Don't just look on the bright side—talk about it

1975, has led many investigators to associate how people think about aging as the key to a longer life. Other studies have given similar results for health status. What people report about their health, that is, "excellent" versus something else—like "terrible," always seems to be a better predictor of actual health than blood pressure readings, cholesterol levels, heart rates and the like. So, the Ohio studies should not be a big surprise. Still, they are of interest, especially if you are getting old, say, over 50.

The Ohio researchers (from Yale University) tracked 660 residents, about half men and half women aged 50 to 94, living in small towns in Ohio. Those with positive attitudes about getting older lasted 7 1/2 years longer than those not so enthused about the prospect. Typical questions explored responses to statements such as, "As you get older, you get less useful." Agree or not? Other examples include, "Are you as happy," and "Do you have as much pep as you had in your younger days?"

What kind of questions were these, anyway? Were these researchers kidding? Of course people get less useful as they get older, if not less happy and "peppy" as the years pass! Did the 94 year-old really and truly think he was more useful and "peppy" now than, let's say, decades ago as a member of an Ohio sports team or business when he was but a mere 50 or so? If he answered that question by stating that he believed he is just as useful now and as peppy as ever, he's either a demented old loon, in deep denial or just having a little fun with the folks conducting the Ohio Longitudinal Study of Aging and Retirement. There could be other reasons for the fact he lived 7 1/2 years (on average) longer than the other 94 year-olds who said, "Of course I get less useful and peppy, and naturally I'm not at all happy about it! Neither is my 25 year-old coed girlfriend!" Or, something like that. For being honest, he has to give up 7 1/2 years? Is that what these Ohio researchers are trying to tell us?

Oh well, in a way this all seems fair enough. Why should the gods, nature or the Grim Reaper harvest those who want to stay around, especially if they are upbeat about having to pay the price of aging (slower 10K times, memory problems, difficulties getting dates, for examples?) Maybe there IS justice in this world, after all.

One of the theories to explain the data is that the survivors with the bright side outlooks simply internalized the good feelings that go with learned optimism from an early age. That upbeat attitude is what served them, not the answers they gave in the surveys. You probably guessed as much. We would all expect folks with better attitudes about getting older (and everything else) to live longer than others less positive about their situations. The key variable, then, might well be a positive, overall optimistic outlook. That's just one more reason to do your best to be well and always look on the bright side of life. Even if you have to fake a bit of optimism about getting older! Sincerity seems to be key; if you can fake that, you'll have it made.

Of course, it's surely better to TRULY feel bright, cheerful, optimistic and so on, but if you can't, you might want to pretend you do! In his studies of old people in Western Australia, Dr. Grant Donovan found an ability to maintain optimism in the face of adversity crucial to survival and "a significant hallmark of mental health." Donovan's work hinted that "accurate" perceptions of self and the world are not as crucial to one's well-being as "overly positive self-evaluations, exaggerated perceptions of mastery and unrealistic optimism!"

Maslow, Erickson and many believed that keeping in touch with reality was essential to mental health. However, reality is a subjective thing. Maybe a positive illusion, rather than an objective view of a grim reality, is preferable. It may be that an individual's PERCEPTION of his/her health status represents reality, whatever the circumstances, and thus is not actually an illusion after all. Perhaps we create our own realities with our beliefs, and the feelings that follow. Norman Cousins, in his landmark book *Anatomy of an Illness*, would agree with this perspective, as would the Dalai Lama.

In a recent commentary, Australian surgeon John Bell cites the Dalai Lama as follows, "The communists took my country, threw me in jail—who was my enemy? My enemy was hatred and anger, my jailor was my friend." Now there's a guy (god?) with a good attitude and, under the circumstances, a healthy view of reality!

So, work on your optimism, even if being optimistic may seem contrary to the facts in the situation. You may live longer—and you'll definitely enjoy yourself and others more.

Daniel C. Dennett was recently quoted in the New York Times as follows: "Nobody is immune to wishful thinking. It takes scientific discipline to protect ourselves from our own credulity, but we've also found ingenious ways to fool ourselves and others. Some of the methods used to exploit these urges are easy to analyze; others take a little more unpacking." ("Show Me the Science," *New York Times*, August 28, 2005.)

Thinking Well, Not Wishfully

Never read anything into a coincidence

I live in the south, where news events usually contain testimonials to divine intervention in all manner of human affairs. It can be positive news (winning a lottery, for instance) or bad news (the house burned down but somebody was rescued)—it won't matter: God will get credit for helping out. Judging from the local papers, God (or Jesus or unnamed angels) is active in Alabama, Georgia, South Carolina and Florida. Anecdotal accounts have "Him" making guest appearances during Hurricane Katrina in New Orleans and Biloxi. (Never mind that he also must have allowed Katrina to make landfall in the first place.)

While the hurricane, the attendant floodwaters and FEMA wreaked havoc on the entire region, God evidently had nothing to do with that. In the South, God is never faulted for the bad stuff. Nobody asks why He stood aside and allowed Satan (in the form of nature) to blow, decimate, devour, rip and plunder. No, the Deity and his agents are credited with the good stuff, like saving someone's photo album. These little favors evidently are signs to the faithful that prove God is compassionate and cool. To the simple folks on the ground talking to reporters, nothing else explains a bright side to the gloom save the hand of the Lord. When these folks say, "Thank you, Jesus," they mean it, literally. If I were a believer living in some godless place, like San Francisco, for example, I would move to a Southern state—I'd want to be in an area where Jesus is most active in human affairs.

I thought about this Southern phenomenon while reading a review of a book called *Beyond Coincidence* by Martin Plimmer and Brian King. (See "The Quirky Moments When Lightning Does Strike Twice," *New York Times*, January 20, 2006). The book is labeled "a collection of stranger-than-fiction anecdotes wrapped loosely in colorful intellectual tissue paper."

A coincidence is defined as "the occurrence of events that happen at the same time by accident but seem to have some connection" (Merriam-Webster Online). Arthur Koestler once referred to uncanny coincidences as "puns of destiny." If everyone in the south read *Beyond Coincidence*, news stories might become less entertaining (not good) but the level of critical thinking would improve by leaps and bounds (good). Here are some interesting excerpts from *Beyond Coincidence*:

- Coincidences are unusual but not mysterious—they are logical outcomes of the laws of chance. Such laws operate strangely in accord with the nature of psychology and mathematics.

- Humans resist the idea that things occur in random fashion, but that does not affect reality, which functions in this manner. A world without "remarkable" coincidences would be much more amazing than the reverse. Plimmer and King: "Something deep in the mind resists the explanations of the statisticians. Evolution may be to blame."

- A poor grasp of statistics explains coincidences that are, in fact, unremarkable. For example, odds against meeting someone else at a party with the same birthday as your own is not 365 to 1. "In a room with just 23 people, the chances that two of them will share the same birthday are better than even."

- "On average, everyone should have a prophetic dream once

every 19 years, and the odds of a double hole-in-one, although apparently staggering at 1.85 billion to 1, ensure that this occurs about once a year."

- The more people in the world, the more coincidences to expect.

I can't recall who said this (I found it in my own notebook, written some time ago for future reference—maybe I made it up!) but it seems to fit this topic. "The extent of uncritical acceptance of nonsense is an unrecognized health hazard. This affliction affects not only the afflicted, but the entire country, in that it leads to grotesque political outcomes, none more strikingly pernicious than the presidency of GWB." I suspect it was Daniel C. Dennett, as part of the opening quote, but the sentiments are mine, as well.

What is really amazing, even miraculous, is that I was planning to write an essay for years on this topic when I came across the one (or two) Dennett quotes and the review of *Beyond Coincidence* by Martin Plimmer and Brian King. I know some may think it's all part of the way things work, but I know better. I think Zeus reached out and made this info available, just for me.

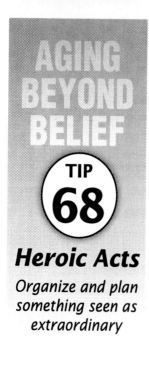

AGING BEYOND BELIEF

TIP 68

Heroic Acts

Organize and plan something seen as extraordinary

*H*eroism means "conduct exhibited in fulfilling a high purpose or attaining a noble end" (*Merriam-Webster Online*). This opens heroism to everyone, including those (like you and me) who may never have occasion to save a life or otherwise act courageously for others in a manner that is daring, risky or otherwise life-threatening. This perspective invites everyone to pursue something personally felt noble and worthy. We can all set high purposes. Who doesn't want to attain something wonderful? Be heroic—consider it and, if you dare, sneak up on whatever it might be, little by little and bit by bit, over time.

At any age, a readiness to perform an act of heroism is a good thing, but it can take on a special consequence for an older person. The latter might have been led to believe that the best of times have passed. Yet, by organizing and acting on a plan for a deed or mission personally deemed heroic, you can eliminate this sense of being over the hill, or believing that you are beyond heroic possibilities. In my view, a heroic mindset will contribute to added confidence, good feelings about the quality of your life and a focus on a worthy future. In summary, just entertaining the possibility of a heroic act will reinforce your resolve to prepare, mentally and physically, for a quality future and thus whatever special challenges may yet come your way.

I think a heroic act or purpose can be anything that meets certain criteria, which include the following:

- Requires extensive preparation, perhaps several months in duration.

- Invites substantial commitment, with a specific outcome in mind that entails consistent training or other preparations.

- Involves no guarantees. You can never be sure of realizing a goal worthy enough to be classed as heroic.

- Inner driven—the focus must be upon meeting your own standards, not qualifying to measure up to someone else's expectations.

It can be exceptionally fulfilling to dwell on heroic possibilities. Thinking heroically does not involve a desire for medals, statues, plaques or other honors bestowed by others. We all have heard and read about heroes as brave individuals who risked their lives for others when they did not have to and those who accomplished amazing things. Nothing wrong with that—we all have our heroes, defined in varied ways. My own include JFK, Lance Armstrong, Carl Sagan, Mark Twain, Paul Kurtz and my two children—for starters. I do not expect perfection of my heroes (though I hasten to add that my kids ARE perfect—but they are the exception!), or that they always function in ways that seem exceptional. Instead, I simply appreciate my heroes for something they represent or accomplished that I deem impressive, admirable or exceptional. Oftentimes, these feats were managed in the face of long odds.

I'm also impressed with anti-heroes, those who challenge some customs and mores of their society. In certain cases, the larger society comes to appreciate their unique contributions, usually after they have passed from the scene. Examples might include Jack Kevorkian, Madalyn Murray O'Hair and Ambrose Bierce. I'm sure you have your own favorites.

So, think about how you might prepare yourself, even late in life, for some kind of heroic act or mission. A quest planned and pursued over time, with your own brand of panache and style, will be its own reward. You will be sustained by an awareness and appreciation of your quiet heroism and more likely to safeguard your passion for a wellness lifestyle all along the way.

AGING BEYOND BELIEF

TIP 69

The Meaning of Life

Think about life's persistent questions, but don't expect absolute answers others will flock to adopt

While there is little consensus on the meaning of life, or even if there IS an overarching, grand inherent meaning applicable to and for all, most would probably agree about what it is NOT. Included in the perceptions that most would agree are NOT the meaning of life would be religious beliefs different from one's own or, on a secular level, activities related to the avoidance of pain or misfortune or the pursuit of pleasure and wealth/creature comforts. Surely there has to be more. Well—what then?

Viktor Frankl and countless existential thinkers have urged a conscious quest for addressing this question. Irving Yalom (author of *Existential Psychotherapy*) suggests it's good mental health to ponder such questions, even if the answer is ultimately unknowable. Frankl fascinated us with accounts of meanings glimpsed under horrific circumstances (Nazi death camps—see *Man's Search for Meaning*), most of us face less daunting obstacles.

You have been at the quest for a lifestyle. Have you resolved the matter to your satisfaction? I'm still open and looking, but like most others, I've arrived at a few points of view on the matter, including these:

1. Life is without inherent meaning—we have to create meaning.

2. It's better to stay open to new possibilities than settle on dogmas and creeds and be done with the matter and closed to new insights.

3. Most people live lives that are reasonably pleasant, have elements of moderate life quality and are shorter than what might be, given better choices. This is a marked improvement

from what the English philosopher Thomas Hobbes thought of things (as expressed about the life of man in nature), namely, life as "solitary, nasty, brutish and short.")

4. Everyone has made decisions about meaning and purpose; unfortunately, many are unaware of their choices or are uncomfortable or resistant to discussing them.

5. The search for meaning and purpose should be continuous, throughout life.

These propositions are just opinions—and as Dennis Miller would add, "I could be wrong about this." Maybe you are more impressed with the observation of Bill Waterson's cartoon character Calvin, whose idea was that, "the meaning of life is people should do what I want!"

You might, but probably not. "Immerse yourself in the river of life and let the questions drift away" are sentiments expressed, with variations, by Yalom, Maslow, Frankl, Durant and other existential thinkers. Entertain the possibility that life is intrinsically unfair and unjust, that there is no escape from pains and sorrows, gloom and doom. It gets grimmer—no matter how deeply you love or how close you are to others, you still face life alone and change alters everything—and then you die.

We can choose an outlook that is rosy, cheerful and almost reverent with awe at the beauty and grandeur of it all. We can wax eloquent about the fabulous fields of grain, trees laden with fruits and seas with a superabundance of nourishing goodies. We can do all this and more, but it's still a good idea to remember that everything out there is eating something, usually smaller, slower or less fearsome than itself.

Make the most of every day. Increase your muscle mass with exercise and a sensible diet. Seek a degree (or two) of peace and harmony. Try to be of service. Find ways to participate where you feel supported and valued. Manage yourself first. Look on the bright side of life.

A Parting Word—or Two

Somebody has to do something,
and it is just incredibly pathetic
that it has to be us.

—Jerry Garcia, Grateful Dead

Americans are not aging well. Nearly two-thirds are too heavy, underfit and over-medicated. Most are way too dependent on physicians, prescriptions and preachers. People are too little resistant to baloney and superstition but overly resistant to science, reason, responsibility and the fine art of living well. In short, things are out of whack and somebody has to do something. What's to be done?

Well, it may indeed be "just incredibly pathetic" but the late, great guitarist of the Grateful Dead was right – "it has to be us."

Thanks for considering 69 different ways for aging well while exercising your inalienable rights to (a high quality of) life, liberty and the pursuit of happiness.

All the best. Please be well.

—Don

#11 -

Printed in the United States
87289LV00005B/1-135/A